DATA INTERPRETATION FOR MEDICAL STUDENTS

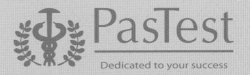

PasTest

Dedicated to your success

DATA INTERPRETATION FOR MEDICAL STUDENTS

Paul Hamilton
BSc(Hons), MB BCh BAO(Hons)
Specialist Registrar in Clinical Pharmacology
and General Internal Medicine
Belfast City Hospital
Belfast

Ian Bickle
MB MCh BAO(Hons)
Specialist Registrar
Radiology
North Trent & Sheffield Training Scheme
Sheffield

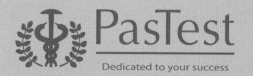

PasTest
Dedicated to your success

© 2006 PASTEST LTD
Egerton Court
Parkgate Estate
Knutsford
Cheshire
WA16 8DX

Telephone: 01565 752000

First published 2006, reprinted 2007, 2008

ISBN: 1 904627 66 8
ISBN: 978 1 904627 66 1

A catalogue record for this book is available from the British Library.

The information contained within this book was obtained by the authors from reliable sources. However, while every effort has been make to ensure its accuracy, no responsibility for loss, damage or injury occasioned to any person acting or refraining from action as a result of information contained herein can be accepted by the publishers or authors.

PasTest Revision Books and Intensive Courses

PasTest has been established in the field of postgraduate medical education since 1972, providing revision books and intensive study courses for doctors preparing for their professional examinations.

Books and courses are available for the following specialties:

MRCGP, MRCP Parts 1 and 2, MRCPCH Parts 1 and 2, MRCPsych, MRCS, MRCOG Parts 1 and 2, DRCOG, DCH, FRCA, PLAB Parts 1 and 2, Dental Students, Dentists and Dental Nurses.

For further details contact:

PasTest, Freepost, Knutsford, Cheshire WA16 7BR

Tel: 01565 752000 Fax: 01565 650264

www.pastest.co.uk enquiries@pastest.co.uk

Illustrations by Ben Stockham
Text prepared by Carnegie Book Production, Lancaster, UK

Printed and bound in the UK by The Alden Group

Contents

Introduction

Data Interpretation for Medical Students has been written not only to help you pass examinations, but to enhance your understanding of the commonly requested tests in medicine. This will hopefully benefit both you and your patients when you become a qualified doctor.

The vast majority of the test results that you will be expected to interpret are included. Related tests have been grouped together in a logical fashion; however, in places, references have been made to other chapters.

The book has been designed very much with ease of use in mind. It can be read from cover to cover. Alternatively, the reader may like to 'dip in and dip out' as necessary. Generally speaking, a discussion is provided to explain the background information relating to a test. You can then assess your understanding by working through the case scenarios at the end of the section or chapter. Detailed answers are provided to ensure that you understand the information. Some sections are short, and do not lend themselves to case scenarios. Aspects of these tests can be found in the complete clinical cases found at the back of the book. These cases are designed to emulate real life, and will test your interpretation of a wide variety of data. At the start of each complete clinical case, we have included a list of the types of data contained therein.

Interpretation of test results requires knowledge of 'normal' values. An extensive list of normal values is found on page viii–xi. We have chosen not to list normal values beside each set of data found throughout the book. This will hopefully encourage you to remember normal values, and will stand you in good stead for working as a doctor, when such values are often not available.

Some points hold true regardless of the type of data being approached. Firstly, if an unexpected result is obtained, always consider the possibility that an error may have been made. Repeating a test will help clarify this issue. Secondly, always interpret a test with a specific clinical context in mind.

We hope that you find this book usable and enjoyable.

PH
IB

Acknowledgements

We have included material which we feel represents common scenarios and that best illustrates the various investigations in medicine. All material has received intensive feedback during the production process to ensure it is readable and usable. We both greatly value constructive criticism, and ideas to improve this text further would be very welcome. Please e-mail us on datainterpretationformedicalstudents@pastest.co.uk if you have any suggestions.

A hugely influential contributor to this book must be mentioned first. Sandy Davey is a current medical student in Queen's University Belfast. His unique qualities, limitless enthusiasm and bravery to comment have helped shape the final draft of this book. We both owe him a huge debt of gratitude.

A special mention must also be made of the contributions of Professor Patrick Bell who reviewed the book critically.

We also owe our Commissioning Editor at Pastest, Elizabeth Kerr, our sincere thanks and apologies – thanks for supporting us throughout this project and making valuable comments; apologies for having to put up with our incessant demands, impatience and peculiarities.

Thanks are extended to Joel Rankin for assisting with the ECGs, Dr Barry Kelly for providing a selection of radiographs, and Dr Ann Johnston for reviewing the neurology section.

PH would like to thank his parents and sister Kerry for their never-ending support and encouragement. He also thanks Anna for her incredible patience during the writing process.

ICB would like to thank Haiza who, despite his spending hours putting this book together, still agreed to marry him!

Normal values

Haematology

Activated Partial Thromboplastin Time (APTT)	35–45 s
Bleeding Time	3–9 min
D-Dimer	<0.5 mg/l
Erythrocyte Sedimentation Rate (ESR)	
Males	0–15 mm/h
Females	0–22 mm/h
Ferritin	12–200 µg/l
Fibrinogen	2–4 g/l
Folate	>2 µg/l
Haemoglobin (Hb)	
Males	13.5–18 g/dl
Females	11.5–16 g/dl
Iron	11–32 mol/l
Mean Cell Volume (MCV)	76–96 fl
Packed Cell Volume (PCV)	
Males	0.4–0.54
Females	0.37–0.47
Platelets	150–400 x 10^9/l
Prothrombin Time (PT)	12–16 s
Red Cell Distribution Width (RDW)	12–15%
Reticulocytes	0.5–2.5% of red blood cells
Total Iron-Binding Capacity (TIBC)	42–80 mol/l
Vitamin B_{12}	>150 ng/l
White Cell Count (WCC)	4.0–11.0 x 10^9/l
Neutrophils	2.0–7.5 x 10^9/l
Lymphocytes	1.5–4.0 x 10^9/l
Eosinophils	0.04–0.4 x 10^9/l
Monocytes	0.2–0.8 x 10^9/l
Basophils	0.0–0.1 x 10^9/l

Biochemistry

Alanine Aminotransferase (ALT)	5–35 IU/l
Albumin	35–50 g/l
Alcohol	Nil
Alkaline Phosphatase (ALP)	30–150 U/l
Alpha Feto-Protein (α–FP)	
<50 years	<10 kU/l
50–70 years	<15 kU/l
70–90 years	<20 kU/l
Amylase	25–125 U/l
Anion Gap	12–16 mmol/l
Arterial partial pressure of carbon dioxide breathing room air ($PaCO_2$)	4.7–6.0 kPa
Arterial partial pressure of oxygen breathing room air (PaO_2)	11–13 kPa
Aspartate Aminotransferase (AST)	5–35 IU/l
Base Excess (BE)	−2 to +2 mmol/l
Beta Human Chorionic Gonadotrophin (β–HCG)	<5 U/l
Bicarbonate (HCO_3-)	24–30 mmol/l
CA–125	<35 U/ml
CA–19–9	<37 U/ml
Calcium (Ca^{2+}) (total)	2.10–2.65 mmol/l
Carboxyhaemoglobin	<5% of total haemoglobin
Carcinoembryonic Antigen (CEA)	<10 ng/ml
Chloride (Cl^-)	95–105 mmol/l
C-Reactive Protein (CRP)	<10 mg/l
Creatine Kinase	
Male	25–195 IU/l
Female	25–170 IU/l
CK–MB	<25 IU/l
Creatinine	79–118 µmol/l (dependent on muscle mass)
Gamma-Glutamyl Transpeptidase (GGT)	
Male	11–58 IU/l
Female	7-33 IU/l
Globulin	18–36 g/l
Glucose	See Page 125
HbA1C	3.8–6.4 %
Lactate	0.5–2.0 mmol/l
Lactate Dehydrogenase (LDH)	70–250 IU/l
Osmolality (Plasma)	280–300 mosmol/kg
Paracetamol	Nil

pH	7.35–7.45
Phosphate (PO_4^{3-})	0.8–1.45 mmol/l
Potassium (K^+)	3.5–5.0 mmol/l
Prostate Specific Antigen (Males)	
40–49 years	<2.5 ng/ml
50–59 years	<3.5 ng/ml
60–69 years	<4.5 ng/ml
70–79 years	<6.5 ng/ml
Salicylates	Nil
Sodium (Na^+)	135–145 mmol/l
Total Bilirubin	3–17 mol/l
Total Protein	60–80 g/l
Troponin I	<0.1 µg/l
Urate	0.15–0.50 mmol/l
Urea	2.5–6.7 mmol/l

Endocrinology

Cortisol	
9 am	200–700 nmol/l
10 pm	50-250 nmol/l
Free thyroxine (T_4)	7.6–19.7 pmol/l
Thyroid stimulating hormone (TSH)	0.4–4.5 mU/l
Total thyroxine (T_4)	70–140 nmol/l

Immunoglobulins

IgA   0.8–4.0 g/l
IgG   7.0–14.5 g/l
IgM   0.45–2.0 g/l

Therapeutic Drug Levels

Digoxin (6 hours post-dose)	1–2 nmol/l
Lithium	0.5–1.5 mmol/l

Cerebrospinal Fluid

Glucose	2.5–4.4 mmol/l (2/3 plasma value)
Red Cell Count (RCC)	0/mm^3
Total Protein	<0.45 g/l
White Cell Count (WCC)	<5/mm^3

Urine

Creatinine Clearance	
Male	85–125 ml/min
Female	75–115 ml/min
Metanephrines	<5.5 μmol/day
Osmolality	250–1250 mosmol/kg
Protein	<0.2 g/day

Sweat

Chloride	<60 mmol/l

HAEMATOLOGY

1

HAEMATOLOGY

Abnormalities with red blood cells

Anaemia

Anaemia describes a low level of haemoglobin. It is usually defined by an arbitrary cut-off haemoglobin concentration (eg 13.5 g/dl in men, 11.5 g/dl in women), below which a patient is deemed to be anaemic.

Anaemia can be split into three big groups by looking at the size of the red blood cells (erythrocytes). In microcytic anaemia red cells are small, in normocytic anaemia they are normal size, and in macrocytic anaemia they are large. The mean cell volume (MCV) provides an average measurement of red cell size.

TYPE OF ANAEMIA	SIZE OF ERYTHROCYTES
Microcytic	Small
Normocytic	Normal
Macrocytic	Large

The diagram on page 4 shows the various causes based on this classification of anaemia.

Note that the MCV provides a measure of average cell size, and this is reliable in most instances. If, however, a patient has two ongoing pathologies, such as iron deficiency and folate deficiency, the MCV can be unreliable. They may have two populations of red cells, one with a low MCV and another with a high MCV. When these measures are averaged, the MCV will be normal. For this reason, the red cell distribution width (RDW) is sometimes measured. This gives an indication of the distribution of red cell sizes. This measure will be raised if two red cell populations are present.

Fig 1.1: The various causes of the major classifications of anaemia.

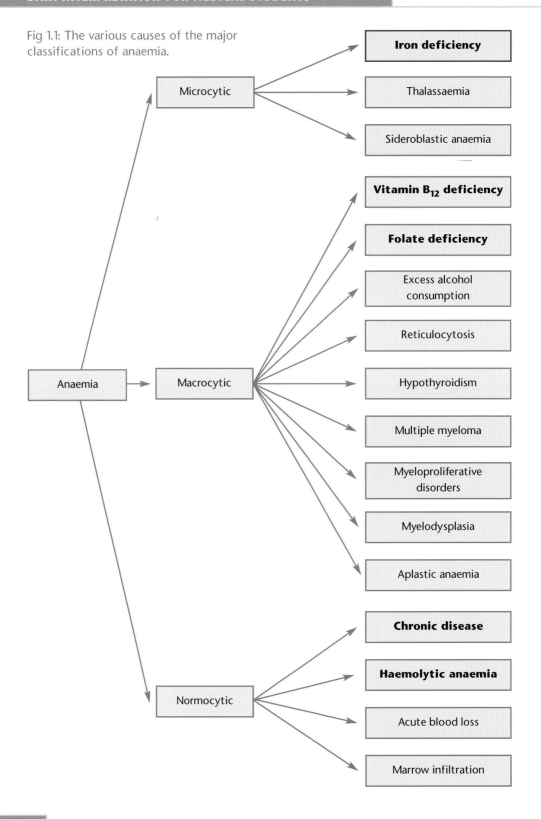

Haematinics

Deficiencies in any of three key nutrients – iron, vitamin B_{12} and folate – can result in anaemia. These nutrients are called haematinics. Iron deficiency is the commonest cause of anaemia, and is commonly found in association with blood loss.

DEFICIENCY	TYPE OF ANAEMIA
Iron	Microcytic
Vitamin B_{12}	Macrocytic
Folate	Macrocytic

Finding a haematinic deficiency is only the first part of establishing the cause of anaemia. Where possible, the cause of the nutrient deficiency should also be sought. For example, iron deficiency is often due to occult blood loss from the gastrointestinal tract, and endoscopy may be employed to search for this.

Knowledge of exactly where haematinics are absorbed from the gastrointestinal tract can sometimes help localise the pathology underlying anaemia. These sites are shown in the box below.

HAEMATINIC	ABSORBED FROM
Iron	Duodenum and jejunum
Vitamin B_{12}	Terminal ileum
Folate	Small bowel

Iron studies

A good understanding of how the body handles iron is required before iron studies can be interpreted.

Iron is best absorbed from the upper small bowel in the ferrous (Fe^{2+}) state. Iron is transported across the intestinal cell and into the plasma. Iron in the plasma is carried to developing red cells in the bone marrow by a protein called transferrin. Iron is stored in the body as ferritin and haemosiderin. Red cells have transferrin receptors (soluble transferrin receptors, sTfR) which can be measured in plasma.

COMPONENTS OF AN IRON PROFILE
Serum iron
Serum total iron-binding capacity (serum TIBC)
Serum ferritin
Serum soluble transferrin receptors

In iron deficiency states, iron studies are as follows:

IRON PARAMETER	RESULT
Serum iron	Reduced
Serum total iron-binding capacity	Increased – the body tries hard to bind any iron around the system
Serum ferritin	Reduced – since iron stores are low
Serum sTfR	Increased – since red cells attempt to absorb any iron in the system

To make matters a little more confusing, ferritin behaves as an acute phase reactant – its level increases with active inflammation, in the same way as the erythrocyte sedimentation rate (ESR) and C reactive protein (CRP) (see pages 15 and 88). This means that, in states of iron deficiency associated with an ongoing inflammatory process (eg an active infection), the serum ferritin level may be high. However, the sTfR will reveal the true state of affairs.

In anaemia of chronic disease, iron studies are commonly as follows:

IRON PARAMETER	RESULT
Serum iron	Normal or slightly reduced
Serum total iron-binding capacity	Reduced
Serum ferritin	May be raised as acute phase reactant
Serum sTfR	Normal – reflecting the true state of body iron levels

In cases of diagnostic uncertainty, a bone marrow biopsy can be obtained and stained for the presence of iron. In iron deficiency states, no iron will be seen in the marrow.

Iron studies are also abnormal in states of iron overload. This is commonly seen in haemochromatosis and in haematological conditions that require frequent blood transfusions. In such cases, serum iron and ferritin are raised. The total iron-binding capacity (TIBC) is usually low.

Vitamin B$_{12}$

Vitamin B$_{12}$ deficiency may result from inadequate intake, but the commonest reason for deficiency relates to poor absorption.

In health, vitamin B$_{12}$ is bound to a protein called intrinsic factor secreted by gastric parietal cells. The vitamin is then absorbed from the ileum. Poor absorption generally results from absence of intrinsic factor or disease of the ileum.

The commonest disease causing vitamin B$_{12}$ deficiency is pernicious anaemia, in which there is defective intrinsic factor production. The disease is associated with autoantibodies against gustic parietal cells and intrinsic factor (see Chapter 8, Immunology).

Schilling test

The Schilling test may be used to distinguish between the various causes of vitamin B$_{12}$ deficiency. In this test, patients are given two doses of vitamin B$_{12}$. One dose is radioactively labelled, and is given orally. The other dose is given intramuscularly with the aim of flushing absorbed radiolabelled vitamin B$_{12}$ into the urine. The urine is collected over a period of 24 h. Normally, a proportion of the oral vitamin B$_{12}$ dose will be absorbed and excreted more than 10% of the oral dose will be excreted in the urine. With vitamin B$_{12}$ malabsorption, this amount will be reduced.

The test is repeated with an oral preparation of intrinsic factor being given at the same time as the oral dose of vitamin B$_{12}$. If the test results are now normal, one can assume that the patient's problem lies with inadequate intrinsic factor. If the test is still abnormal, the problem most likely lies in the ileum.

One possible cause of ileal disease is bacterial overgrowth. In order to test for this possibility, the patient can be given a course of antibiotics. If the Schilling test returns to normal after this, the diagnosis of bacterial overgrowth can be made. Alternatively, bacterial overgrowth can be diagnosed using a breath test. The most commonly used test is the hydrogen breath test. A carbohydrate load is given orally. Bacteria in the small bowel metabolise the carbohydrate, liberating hydrogen which is absorbed and detected in exhaled air.

Folate

Folate analysis is simple. Serum folate levels are measured with a deficiency identified if levels are low.

Haemolytic anaemia

There are many causes of haemolytic anaemia, but in each case there is abnormal destruction of red blood cells.

Evidence of haemolysis

When red blood cells are destroyed, haemoglobin is degraded, and bibirubin liberated. Bilirubin is conjugated in the liver and passed into the bowel in the bile. Here, it is converted into urobilinogen. Some of this is passed in the stools; some is re-absorbed, and excreted in the urine. In cases of haemolysis, the plasma unconjugated bilirubin will rise, and increased amounts of urobilinogen will be detected in the urine. The level of lactate dehydrogenase (LDH) will also rise.

When red cells are destroyed inside blood vessels, haemoglobin is released. Haptoglobins bind to free haemoglobin and escort it to the liver. However, haptoglobins can become saturated and in such circumstances haemoglobin may be passed in the urine (haemoglobinuria), or converted to haemosiderin which is then passed in the urine (haemosiderinuria). Alternatively, further reactions can occur which result in the presence of methaemalbumin in the circulation.

INTRAVASCULAR HAEMOLYSIS IS SUGGESTED BY

- low haptoglobins
- haemosiderinuria
- methaemalbumin (detected in Schumm's test)

With excessive red cell destruction, the bone marrow works hard to replace the number of circulating cells. The number of primitive red cells (reticulocytes) in the circulation therefore increases.

The causes of haemolytic anaemia are illustrated in the diagram on page 9.

Fig 1.2: The causes of haemolytic anaemia.

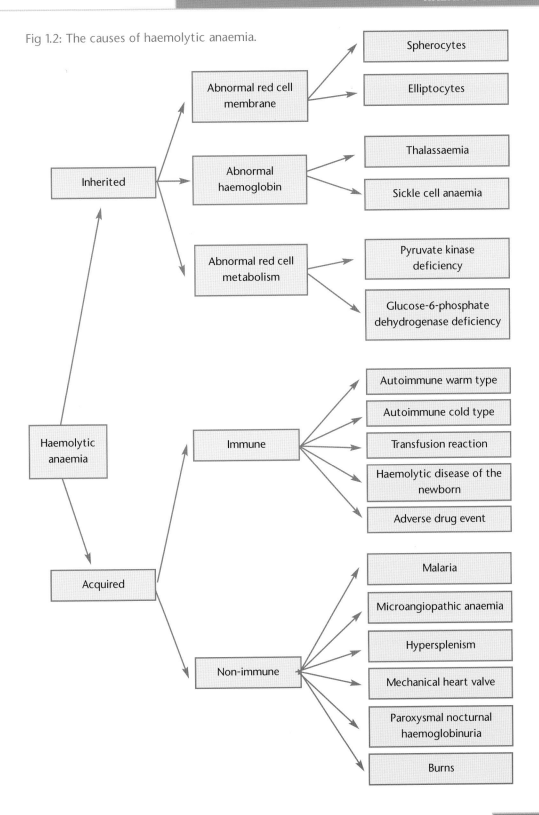

Osmotic fragility test

Hereditary spherocytosis is a condition associated with an abnormal red blood cell membrane where red cells become spherical in shape. The cells are less resilient to damage in this condition. This can be assessed using an osmotic fragility test. Spherocytes have increased osmotic fragility.

Direct antiglobulin test

In autoimmune haemolytic anaemias, antibodies attack red cells and cause their destruction. The main laboratory test for autoimmune haemolytic anaemia is the direct antiglobulin test (DAT or Coombs' test). In this test, antibodies to human immunoglobulin are added to a sample of red cells from the patient. If the red cells are coated in antibodies (ie if the patient has an autoimmune haemolytic anaemia), they will agglutinate.

Polycythaemia

Polycythaemia is defined as a packed cell volume (PCV) greater than 0.51 in males or greater than 0.48 in females.

POLYCYTHAEMIA
Males – PCV >0.51
Females – PCV >0.48

Red cell mass

In order to distinguish between true and apparent polycythaemia, the red cell mass must be measured. In true polycythaemia, the red cell mass is raised. Apparent polycythaemia is due to a reduction in plasma volume rather than an increase in red cell mass.

Red cell mass is measured by labelling red cells with a radioactive isotope. A predicted red cell mass can be calcuated based on the patient's height and weight. True polycythaemia is diagnosed if the red cell mass is more than 25% higher than that predicted.

To distinguish between causes of true polycythaemia, further tests should be arranged. These usually include:

- arterial blood gas analysis (to look for hypoxia)
- erythropoietin level (to detect inappropriately high levels)
- an ultrasound of the abdomen (to detect structural renal or hepatic disease and to visualise the spleen)
- further investigations depending on the most likely cause.

Polycythaemia can be subdivided as shown in the diagram below.

Fig 1.3: Causes of polycythaemia.

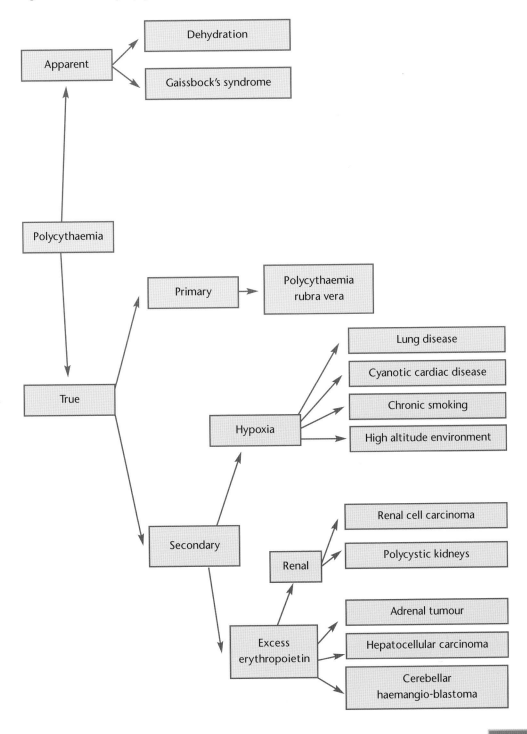

Abnormalities with white blood cells

Abnormal white cell counts

Abnormalities in white blood cell counts are common. The most frequently occurring abnormalities are listed in the boxes below with common causes.

COMMON CAUSES OF NEUTROPHILIA (NEUTROPHILS >7.5 X 10^9/l)

Bacterial infections	Malignancy
Inflammation	Myeloproliferative disorders
Necrosis, eg after myocardial infarction	Metabolic disorders, eg renal failure
Treatment with corticosteroids	

COMMON CAUSES OF NEUTROPENIA (NEUTROPHILS <2.0 X 10^9/l)

Post-chemotherapy
Post-radiotherapy
Adverse drug reactions, eg clozapine, carbimazole
Viral infection
Felty's syndrome

COMMON CAUSES OF LYMPHOCYTOSIS (LYMPHOCYTES >3.5 X 10^9/l)

Viral infections
Chronic infections, eg TB
Chronic lymphocytic leukaemia
Lymphomas

COMMON CAUSES OF EOSINOPHILIA (EOSINOPHILS >0.5 X 10^9/l)

Allergic disorders	Skin diseases, eg eczema
Parasite infection	Malignancy, eg Hodgkin's disease
Hypereosinophilic syndrome	Allergic bronchopulmonary aspergillosis

Abnormalities with platelets

Thrombocytosis

Thrombocytosis describes a high platelet count (>400 x 10^9/l). The common causes are shown in the box below.

COMMON CAUSES OF THROMBOCYTOSIS	
Primary haematological diseases:	**Reactive thrombocytosis secondary to:**
• Essential thrombocythaemia and other myeloproliferative disorders • Chronic myeloid leukaemia • Myelodysplasia	• Infection • Inflammation • Malignancy • Bleeding • Pregnancy • Post-splenectomy

Thrombocytopenia

Thrombocytopenia describes a low platelet count (<150 x 10^9/l). The common causes are shown in the box below.

CAUSES OF THROMBOCYTOPENIA

Reduced platelet production due to bone marrow failure:
• Infections (particularly viral, eg infectious mononucleosis)
• Drug induced, eg penicillamine
• Leukaemia
• Aplastic anaemia
• Myelofibrosis (later stages)
• Bone marrow replacement with tumour, eg myeloma or metastases
• Myelodysplasia
• Megaloblastic anaemia
 	
Increased platelet destruction:
• Immune-mediated platelet destruction
  • Autoimmune idiopathic thrombocytopenia purpura (AITP)
  • Drug induced, particularly heparin-induced thrombocytopenia (HIT)
• Hypersplenism
• Thrombotic thrombocytopenic purpura/haemolytic uraemic syndrome
• Disseminated intravascular coagulation (DIC)
• After a massive blood transfusion

Pancytopenia

Pancytopenia is the term used to describe the pattern present when there are low levels of red blood cells, white blood cells and platelets in the circulation. There are a wide variety of causes, the most common of which are shown in the box.

COMMON CAUSES OF PANCYTOPENIA

- Aplastic anaemia
- Bone marrow infiltration, eg with tumour
- Hypersplenism
- Megaloblastic anaemia
- Sepsis
- Systemic lupus erythematosis (SLE)

Erythrocyte sedimentation rate (ESR)

The erythrocyte sedimentation rate (ESR) measures how rapidly red blood cells form sediment when a column of blood is kept upright for 1 h. The further the red cells sink in the hour, the higher the ESR.

The ESR is a non-specific marker of disease. In inflammatory processes, raised levels of plasma proteins result in red blood cells forming clumps called rouleaux. These clumps of cells sink more easily than single cells, and thus, in the presence of such proteins, the ESR is high.

The ESR normally rises with advancing age, but levels of more than 35 mm/h should raise the suspicion of a disease process in any age group. Causes of a raised ESR are myriad. Common examples are listed in the box below.

COMMON CAUSES OF A RAISED ESR

- Infectious disease
- Neoplastic disease (particularly multiple myeloma)
- Connective tissue disease (particularly giant cell arteritis and polymyalgia rheumatica)
- Anaemia
- Renal disease

Blood film abnormalities

Examination of a peripheral blood film can aid or clinch a diagnosis in a range of clinical scenarios. Correct identification of various cell types requires significant training, but knowledge of the different terminology used can greatly aid interpretation of blood film reports. The following abnormal cell types are among those most commonly seen.

Abnormal erythrocyte colour or shape

ABNORMALITY	FOUND IN
Hypochromic cells	Iron deficiency or defective haemoglobin synthesis
Microcytosis	Iron deficiency or defective haemoglobin synthesis
Macrocytosis	Megaloblastic anaemia, high alcohol intake, liver disease
Pencil cells	Iron deficiency
Spherocytes	Hereditary spherocytosis, haemolytic anaemia, burns
Elliptocytes	Hereditary elliptocytosis, thalassaemia major, iron deficiency
Acanthocytes	Abetalipoproteinaemia, post-splenectomy, liver disease
Target cells	Thalassaemia, iron deficiency, post-splenectomy, liver disease
Stomatocytes	Hereditary stomatocytosis, high alcohol intake, liver disease
Ecchinocytes	Post-splenectomy, liver disease
Sickle cells	Sickle cell anaemia (homozygous HbS disease)
Fragmented cells	Microangiopathic haemolytic anaemia, haemolytic uraemic syndrome, thrombotic thrombocytopenic purpura, mechanical heart valves, disseminated intravascular coagulation
Burr cells	Microangiopathic haemolytic anaemia, uraemia, pyruvate kinase deficiency
Tear cells (dacryocytes)	Myelofibrosis and other causes of extramedullary haematopoiesis
Poikilocytosis	Iron deficiency
Anisochromia	Iron deficiency

Abnormalities inside erythrocytes

ABNORMALITY	FOUND IN
Heinz bodies	Unstable haemoglobin states
Howell–Jolly bodies	Hyposplenism, post-splenectomy
Pappenheimer bodies	Post-splenectomy, haemolytic anaemia, sideroblastic anaemia
Basophilic stippling	Iron poisoning, thalassaemia, myelodysplasia
Cabot's rings	Myelodysplasia, megaloblastic anaemia

Abnormal white blood cells

ABNORMALITY	FOUND IN
Hypersegmented neutrophils	Megaloblastic anaemias, chronic infections
Toxic granulation of neutrophils	Bacterial infection, poisoning, burns, chemotherapy
Auer rods	Acute myeloid leukaemia

Leukoerythroblastic blood film

This is a term used to describe the overall appearance of a blood film in which immature red and white blood cells are seen in peripheral blood. There are several causes.

CAUSES OF A LEUKOERYTHROBLASTIC BLOOD FILM
• Bone marrow infiltration, eg with tumour • Idiopathic myelofibrosis • Severe sepsis • Haemolysis

Coagulation disorders

Haemostasis (the process of stopping bleeding) is a complex process. It involves the interplay of blood vessel walls, platelets and clotting factors. The common tests used to assess coagulation are as follows:

COMMON TESTS OF COAGULATION
• Prothrombin time (PT) • International normalised ratio (INR) • Activated partial thromboplastin time (APTT) • Bleeding time

Prothrombin time

The PT is dependent on clotting factors I, II, V, VII and X. In clinical practice, it is most commonly measured to assess the synthetic function of the liver (eg in liver failure), or to monitor the effects of warfarin therapy.

International normalised ratio

To allow comparison of coagulation results between laboratories, the PT is often converted to the INR, by applying a correction factor. This takes into account differences in laboratory materials, and means that the patient's INR should be the same regardless of the laboratory used to measure it.

The INR is the parameter most commonly used to monitor the effects of warfarin. In a patient with normal coagulation, the INR will be close to 1.0 before warfarin is commenced. As warfarin is introduced, the INR rises. The higher the INR, the less coagulable the blood becomes (ie the more difficult it will be for the blood to clot). Target INRs are set, and warfarin dosing must be adjusted to aim for these targets.

DISEASE	TARGET INR
Deep venous thrombosis (DVT)	2.5
Pulmonary embolism (PE)	2.5
Atrial fibrillation	2.5
Mechanical prosthetic heart valve	2.5
Recurrent DVT/PE in a patient with a therapeutic INR	3.5

The essence of warfarin prescribing involves increasing the dose if the INR is too low, reducing the dose if the INR is too high, and omitting it if the INR is dangerously high or the patient is bleeding. An example of a warfarin prescribing chart is shown on page 366.

Activated partial thromboplastin time

The APTT depends on all clotting factors except factor VII. In clinical practice, the APTT is used most commonly in patients receiving an infusion of heparin. The APTT is monitored frequently, and the rate of the heparin infusion adjusted to achieve the desired level of anticoagulation. With the common prescribing of molecular weight heparin, this process is uncommonly undertaken. A frequent cause of concern relates to elevated APTTs in patients with central venous catheters. The proximal end of such catheters are often filled with heparin to keep the lumens patent when they are not being used. A spuriously high APTT will be obtained if blood is withdrawn from one such lumen. If the APTT is tested on a sample of blood tested peripherally, the true value will be obtained.

Coagulation correction testing

In cases of deranged coagulation, laboratories will often perform a coagulation correction test. This is performed to detect problems in coagulation arising because of a low level of a particular clotting factor. In essence, normal plasma (containing normal clotting factors) is mixed with the patient's sample. If the patient is deficient in clotting factors, a deranged coagulation profile would be expected to normalise. There will be no change, however, if an inhibitor of coagulation is present. Specialised assays for individual clotting factors are also available.

Bleeding time

Bleeding time is measured directly at the bed-side. A sphygmomanometer cuff is inflated around the patient's arm to 40 mmHg. A specially designed blade is then used to make a small puncture in the arm. Blood is removed from the area at fixed time intervals (eg 15 s) using a piece of filter paper to soak it up. The time taken for bleeding to stop is recorded. Elevated bleeding times indicate defective platelet function or low platelet numbers. This test should not be performed if the patient is known to have severe thrombocytopenia.

Bear in mind that patients with abnormal numbers or deranged function of platelets may also have abnormal bleeding. Patients with von Willebrand's disease may have normal coagulation profiles.

DON'T FORGET

Patients with von Willebrand's disease may have normal coagulation profiles

Disseminated intravascular coagulation

Disseminated intravascular coagulation (DIC) is a disease of two apparently conflicting problems. On the one hand, fibrin deposition in various organs results in areas of micro-infarction. On the other hand, the body's supplies of clotting factors become used up because of all the clotting, leaving the patient prone to bleeding.

DISSEMINATED INTRAVASCULAR COAGULATION

A disease in which clotting and bleeding cause problems simultaneously

Typical laboratory findings in DIC are as follows:

Raised PT and APTT	Since clotting factors are reduced
Reduced fibrinogen	Due to widespread fibrin formation
Raised D-dimer	Due to the body's attempt to break down the excess fibrin deposits

D-dimer

D-dimer is the most commonly measured fibrinogen/fibrin degeneration product. It is detected following clot formation in the vasculature, as the body's fibrinolytic system attempts to break them down. D-dimer levels are often tested in cases of suspected deep venous thromboses and pulmonary emboli, and in the majority of cases will be raised. However, D-dimer levels are also raised with many other conditions, and a raised level should always be interpreted in light of the clinical scenario.

Case 1

A 48-year-old retired civil servant is concerned with her pale colour and feelings of faintness that have occurred over the past 4 weeks. She had felt well prior to this and enjoyed regular trips to southern France. Brief clinical examination reveals pallor. Her blood tests come to your attention.

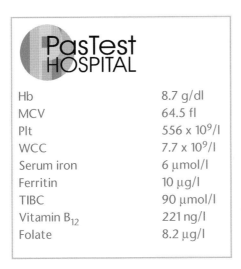

Hb	8.7 g/dl
MCV	64.5 fl
Plt	556 x 10^9/l
WCC	7.7 x 10^9/l
Serum iron	6 μmol/l
Ferritin	10 μg/l
TIBC	90 μmol/l
Vitamin B$_{12}$	221 ng/l
Folate	8.2 μg/l

1. **How would you interpret these results?**

2. **How would you proceed with investigation?**

Answer 1

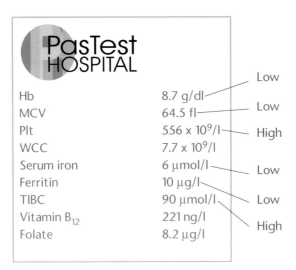

PasTest
HOSPITAL

Hb	8.7 g/dl	Low
MCV	64.5 fl	Low
Plt	556 x 10^9/l	High
WCC	7.7 x 10^9/l	
Serum iron	6 µmol/l	Low
Ferritin	10 µg/l	
TIBC	90 µmol/l	Low
Vitamin B$_{12}$	221 ng/l	
Folate	8.2 µg/l	High

1. This patient has a microcytic anaemia. His iron profile is in keeping with iron deficiency with a low iron, low ferritin and high TIBC. There is a mild thrombocytosis which may indicate active bleeding.

2. The commonest cause for these findings in young women is menorrhagia. In an older female or male, investigations should be carried out to exclude a sinister cause – in particular an occult gastrointestinal tract malignancy. Investigations should begin with a thorough history and clinical examination which should include rectal examination. The next line of investigation usually involves gastrointestinal tract endoscopy and/or barium enema.

Case 2

A 57-year-old woman attends her GP complaining of tiredness. The GP knows her medical history well as she also suffers from Graves' disease. A full blood count was analysed as well as haematinics.

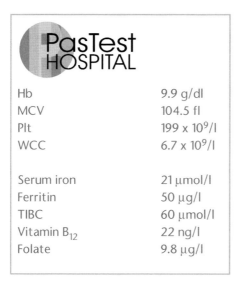

Hb	9.9 g/dl
MCV	104.5 fl
Plt	199 x 10^9/l
WCC	6.7 x 10^9/l
Serum iron	21 μmol/l
Ferritin	50 μg/l
TIBC	60 μmol/l
Vitamin B$_{12}$	22 ng/l
Folate	9.8 μg/l

1.   Interpret these blood results.

Following these results the GP also requests another test shown below.

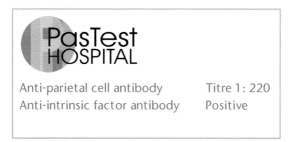

Anti-parietal cell antibody	Titre 1 : 220
Anti-intrinsic factor antibody	Positive

2.   What is the diagnosis?

Answer 2

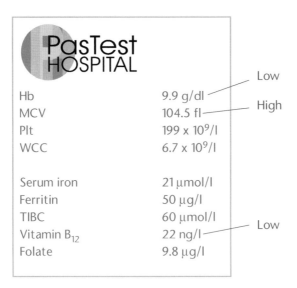

PasTest
HOSPITAL

		Low
Hb	9.9 g/dl	
MCV	104.5 fl	High
Plt	199 x 10^9/l	
WCC	6.7 x 10^9/l	
Serum iron	21 µmol/l	
Ferritin	50 µg/l	
TIBC	60 µmol/l	
Vitamin B$_{12}$	22 ng/l	Low
Folate	9.8 µg/l	

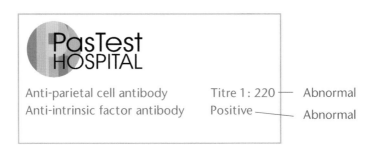

PasTest
HOSPITAL

| Anti-parietal cell antibody | Titre 1: 220 | Abnormal |
| Anti-intrinsic factor antibody | Positive | Abnormal |

1. The haemoglobin is low with an elevated mean cell volume. This patient has a macrocytic anaemia. Haematinics show a low vitamin B$_{12}$ level. Iron studies and folate level are within normal limits.

2. The positive antibodies to gastric parietal cells and intrinsic factor indicate that the likely underlying cause of the anaemia is pernicious anaemia. You will note that the patient was already known to have an autoimmune disease – Graves' disease. Always remember that patients with one autoimmune disease are prone to developing another.

A Schilling test would have been useful in this case. The initial test would show low levels of radiolabelled vitamin B$_{12}$ in the urine. Once the patient was given oral intrinsic factor, urine vitamin B$_{12}$ excretion would be expected to return to normal.

Case 3

A 49-year-old woman with systemic sclerosis complains of malaise and palpitations. Her disease has been quiescent for 2 years and she is not on any immunosuppressant medications. She has a balanced diet and has had no previous surgery. Her rheumatologist requests the following tests:

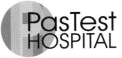
PasTest
HOSPITAL

Hb	8.2 g/dl
MCV	109.4 fl
Plt	169 x 10^9/l
WCC	6.2 x 10^9/l

Serum iron	23 μmol/l
Ferritin	49 μg/l
TIBC	62 μmol/l
Vitamin B$_{12}$	31 ng/l
Folate	>10 μg/l

| Anti-parietal cell antibody | Titre < 1 : 120 |
| Anti-intrinsic factor antibody | Negative |

Schilling test   Without oral intrinsic factor: 0.03 μg radioactive vitamin B$_{12}$ in 24-h urine sample (3% of oral dose)
With oral intrinsic factor: 0.03 μg radioactive vitamin B$_{12}$ in 24-h urine sample (3% of oral dose)

Hydrogen breath test   Early peak in hydrogen excretion

1. **What would you infer from these results?**

2. **What is the reason for performing a hydrogen breath test?**

Answer 3

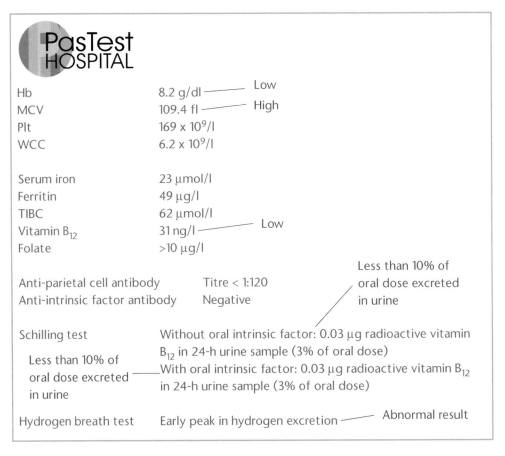

PasTest
HOSPITAL

Hb	8.2 g/dl	Low
MCV	109.4 fl	High
Plt	169 x 10^9/l	
WCC	6.2 x 10^9/l	

Serum iron	23 µmol/l	
Ferritin	49 µg/l	
TIBC	62 µmol/l	
Vitamin B$_{12}$	31 ng/l	Low
Folate	>10 µg/l	

Anti-parietal cell antibody   Titre < 1:120   Less than 10% of
Anti-intrinsic factor antibody   Negative   oral dose excreted
                                                         in urine

Schilling test   Without oral intrinsic factor: 0.03 µg radioactive vitamin
                        B$_{12}$ in 24-h urine sample (3% of oral dose)
  Less than 10% of   With oral intrinsic factor: 0.03 µg radioactive vitamin B$_{12}$
  oral dose excreted   in 24-h urine sample (3% of oral dose)
  in urine

Hydrogen breath test   Early peak in hydrogen excretion ——— Abnormal result

1. This patient has a macrocytic anaemia. Vitamin B$_{12}$ is the only deficient haematinic, but the autoantibodies for pernicious anaemia are negative. The history states that the diet is balanced and no surgery has taken place on the bowel to interfere with the absorption of vitamin B$_{12}$. The Schilling test is abnormal. Normally, at least 10% of the oral dose of radiolabelled vitamin B$_{12}$ is excreted in the urine. In this case, the excreted dose is low, and supplementation with intrinsic factor makes no difference. The likely pathology is therefore in the ileum.

2. The abnormal hydrogen breath test result points to the cause of anaemia – small bowel bacterial overgrowth. Patients with systemic sclerosis are prone to developing this condition. Definitive testing for bacterial overgrowth involves culturing small bowel contents. One would expect a normal Schilling test after an adequate course of appropriate antibiotics.

Case 4

A 34-year-old accountant with a 15-year history of Crohn's disease attends for outpatient review. He feels reasonable, although has not yet been able to hold down full employment after numerous hospital admissions and surgery over the past 10 years. His last surgery involved small bowel resection and anastomosis after further failure of medical therapy. The SHO in the clinic requests the following tests.

PasTest HOSPITAL

Hb	8.9 g/dl
MCV	94.5 fl
Plt	$399 \times 10^9/l$
WCC	$9.7 \times 10^9/l$
RDW	20%
Serum iron	9 μmol/l
Ferritin	10 μg/l
TIBC	80 μmol/l
Vitamin B_{12}	12 ng/l
Folate	1.8 μg/l

What is your interpretation of these tests?

Answer 4

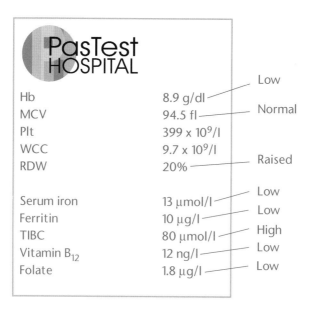

PasTest
HOSPITAL

Hb	8.9 g/dl	Low
MCV	94.5 fl	Normal
Plt	399 x 10⁹/l	
WCC	9.7 x 10⁹/l	
RDW	20%	Raised
Serum iron	13 µmol/l	Low
Ferritin	10 µg/l	Low
TIBC	80 µmol/l	High
Vitamin B₁₂	12 ng/l	Low
Folate	1.8 µg/l	Low

This man has a normocytic anaemia. He is deficient in iron, vitamin B_{12} and folate. The red cell distribution width (RDW) is raised, indicating a wide variation in the size of circulating red cells. The patient is likely to have a dimorphic blood picture, with small red cells resulting from iron deficiency, and large cells resulting from deficiencies of vitamin B_{12} and folate. Crohn's disease is an inflammatory bowel disease involving the whole gastrointestinal tract so has the potential to cause deficiencies in all three haematinics. In this case, multiple operations have left him with a very short small bowel.

Case 5

A 55-year-old woman with essential hypertension attends the medical clinic. Her blood pressure remains elevated despite treatment with four drugs. Her Consultant commences her on methyldopa. Four weeks later she attends the accident and emergency department feeling generally unwell. The A&E doctor sends off a variety of blood tests, which are shown here.

PasTest HOSPITAL

Hb	9.2 g/dl
MCV	93.4 fl
Plt	376 x 10^9/l
WCC	7.2 x 10^9/l
Serum iron	25 µmol/l
Ferritin	154 µg/l
TIBC	65 µmol/l
Vitamin B$_{12}$	198 ng/l
Folate	6.5 µg/l
Total bilirubin	45 µmol/l
AST	25 IU/l
ALT	22 IU/l
GGT	15 IU/l
ALP	98 U/l

She is admitted to the medical unit, and several other tests are requested.

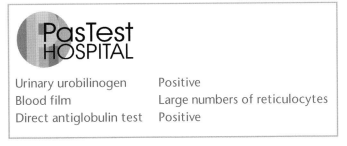

PasTest HOSPITAL

Urinary urobilinogen	Positive
Blood film	Large numbers of reticulocytes
Direct antiglobulin test	Positive

1. **Interpret the results above**

2. **What is the likely diagnosis?**

Answer 5

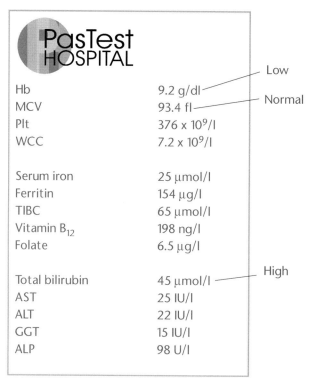

Hb	9.2 g/dl	Low
MCV	93.4 fl	Normal
Plt	376 x 10⁹/l	
WCC	7.2 x 10⁹/l	
Serum iron	25 μmol/l	
Ferritin	154 μg/l	
TIBC	65 μmol/l	
Vitamin B₁₂	198 ng/l	
Folate	6.5 μg/l	
Total bilirubin	45 μmol/l	High
AST	25 IU/l	
ALT	22 IU/l	
GGT	15 IU/l	
ALP	98 U/l	

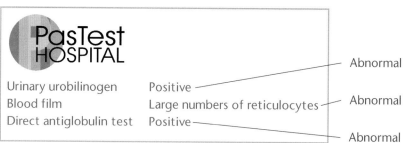

Urinary urobilinogen	Positive	Abnormal
Blood film	Large numbers of reticulocytes	Abnormal
Direct antiglobulin test	Positive	Abnormal

1. This patient has a normocytic anaemia. Her haematinics are normal. She has a raised blood bilirubin level and urobilinogen in the urine which would be in keeping with haemoglobin breakdown. Her blood film shows a reticulocytosis indicating that the bone marrow is working hard to make new red blood cells. The direct antiglobulin test is positive indicating that the patient's red cells are coated with antibodies.

2. The patient has an autoimmune haemolytic anaemia, which is most likely to be an adverse effect of treatment with methyldopa.

Case 6

When on elective in Malawi, you are asked to see a patient. He is 35 years old and complains of anorexia and abdominal discomfort. Examination is unremarkable. A full blood picture is requested.

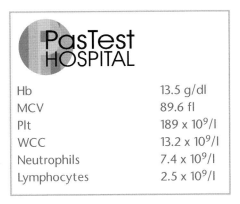

Hb	13.5 g/dl
MCV	89.6 fl
Plt	189 x 10^9/l
WCC	13.2 x 10^9/l
Neutrophils	7.4 x 10^9/l
Lymphocytes	2.5 x 10^9/l

What is the likely diagnosis?

Answer 6

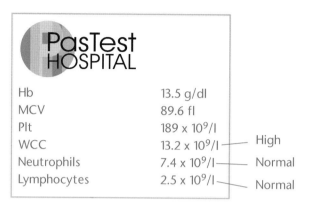

PasTest
HOSPITAL

Hb	13.5 g/dl
MCV	89.6 fl
Plt	189 x 10⁹/l
WCC	13.2 x 10⁹/l — High
Neutrophils	7.4 x 10⁹/l — Normal
Lymphocytes	2.5 x 10⁹/l — Normal

This question is a little sneaky. The key to finding the answer is to remember that the total WCC is equal to the sum of the component parts of the differential white cell count.

DON'T FORGET

Total white cell count = neutrophil count + lympocyte count + eosinophil count + monocyte count + basophil count

In this case, the neutrophil count and lympocyte count together cannot account for the total white cell count ($(7.4 \times 10^9/l) + (2.5 \times 10^9/l) < 13.2 \times 10^9/l$)). There must be a further type of white blood cell in elevated numbers. It is impossible to tell for certain what this cell type might be. However, the likely diagnosis here is helminthic (worm) infection. A full differential white cell count would reveal a raised level of eosinophils.

Case 7

You see a 64-year-old woman in A&E. She has severe chronic obstructive pulmonary disease (COPD), and has been an inpatient on several occasions in the past year. She appears short of breath, and complains of a worsening cough productive of green sputum. This has become worse over the last 3 days. Part of her admission blood tests are shown.

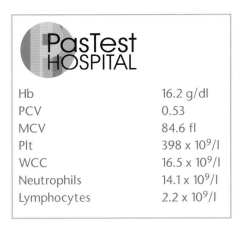

PasTest HOSPITAL	
Hb	16.2 g/dl
PCV	0.53
MCV	84.6 fl
Plt	398 x 10^9/l
WCC	16.5 x 10^9/l
Neutrophils	14.1 x 10^9/l
Lymphocytes	2.2 x 10^9/l

Outline the abnormalities shown, and discuss their most likely causes.

Answer 7

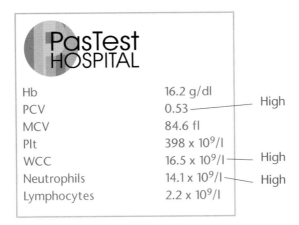

Hb	16.2 g/dl	
PCV	0.53	High
MCV	84.6 fl	
Plt	$398 \times 10^9/l$	
WCC	$16.5 \times 10^9/l$	High
Neutrophils	$14.1 \times 10^9/l$	High
Lymphocytes	$2.2 \times 10^9/l$	

The first abnormality relates to the raised packed cell volume (PCV) indicating polycythaemia. The most likely cause in this case is a true polycythaemia secondary to chronic hypoxia resulting from COPD. Useful tests to confirm this would be an estimation of red cell mass to confirm true polycythaemia, and an arterial blood gas sample to demonstrate hypoxaemia.

The second abnormality relates to the elevated white cell count. Note that the neutrophil count is markedly elevated, and that the sum of the neutrophil and lymphocyte counts almost adds up to the total white cell count. The small discrepancy is due to the presence of a small number of other white blood cells (eosinophils, monocytes and basophils) in the circulation. The most likely cause for this picture is a bacterial infection of the lower respiratory tract.

Case 8

A 74-year-old man presents to the A&E department after a 5 min episode of loss of vision affecting the right eye. Further questioning revealed that the patient had a similar episode 2 days previously. On each occasion the vision was lost rapidly, 'like a curtain being drawn' over the visual field. Direct questioning revealed that he had been lethargic for several weeks, and experienced some pain in his jaw on chewing. Initial blood tests revealed the following:

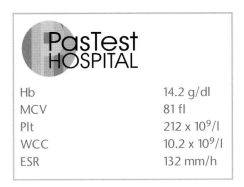

Hb	14.2 g/dl
MCV	81 fl
Plt	212 x 10^9/l
WCC	10.2 x 10^9/l
ESR	132 mm/h

1. **What is the likely diagnosis?**

2. **What treatment would you prescribe immediately?**

Answer 8

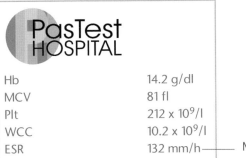

Hb	14.2 g/dl
MCV	81 fl
Plt	212 x 10⁹/l
WCC	10.2 x 10⁹/l
ESR	132 mm/h——— Marked elevation

1. The episode of loss of vision is typical of amaurosis fugax. Taken together with the history of lethargy and jaw pain on eating (jaw claudication), the clinical suspicion must be of temporal arteritis. Such patients are at high risk of complications, including blindness. The extremely high ESR measured here would support this diagnosis. Temporal arteritis is one of the few causes of an ESR greater than 100 mm/h.

2. Treatment should be given rapidly, and should comprise high-dose prednisolone (eg 60–80 mg orally immediately), followed by a reducing dose regimen.

Case 9

You are the junior doctor on the vascular surgical unit. One of your patients, a 75-year-old man with peripheral vascular disease, is due to undergo bypass vascular surgery on his legs. You request a battery of preoperative blood tests. The following results give the nursing staff some concern.

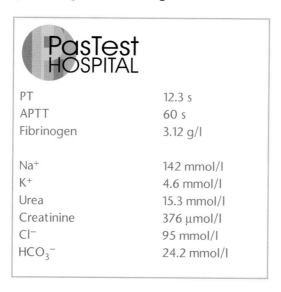

PasTest
HOSPITAL

PT	12.3 s
APTT	60 s
Fibrinogen	3.12 g/l
Na^+	142 mmol/l
K^+	4.6 mmol/l
Urea	15.3 mmol/l
Creatinine	376 µmol/l
Cl^-	95 mmol/l
HCO_3^-	24.2 mmol/l

What should you do next?

Answer 9

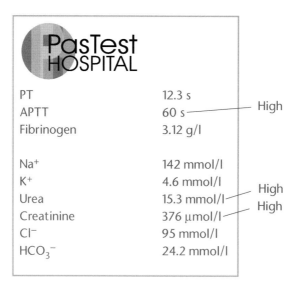

This situation is a common cause for concern. The details omitted from the history above are that the patient has chronic renal failure, and receives haemodialysis three times per week via his indwelling central venous catheter. The raised urea and creatinine are a reflection of the chronic renal failure in this case (see Chapter 2, Biochemistry, for more information).

The cause of the deranged coagulation is most likely because blood has been drawn from the central venous catheter, which is often flushed with a heparin solution. The next step should be to repeat the coagulation profile using blood taken from a peripheral vein.

Case 10

A 58-year-old patient with immunodeficiency is admitted to the intensive care unit with severe pneumonia. Despite aggressive antibiotic therapy, his condition does not improve. On his third day in the unit, the nurses report that he is beginning to bleed around the sites of his indwelling venous lines. The doctor in charge requests a coagulation profile. The blood is taken from a peripheral vein.

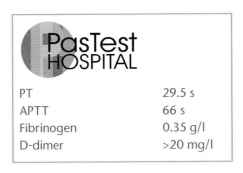

PT	29.5 s
APTT	66 s
Fibrinogen	0.35 g/l
D-dimer	>20 mg/l

What is the likely diagnosis?

Answer 10

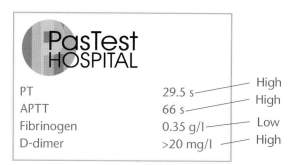

PT	29.5 s	High
APTT	66 s	High
Fibrinogen	0.35 g/l	Low
D-dimer	>20 mg/l	High

The PT and APTT are raised suggesting a tendency to bleed. The fibrinogen level is low indicating that fibrinogen has been used up. The D-dimer level is markedly raised indicating that the body's fibrinolytic system is working hard to disperse clots.

This pattern of abnormalities is typical of DIC, a not uncommon complication in patients with critical illness. Blood product support will be required, and the advice of a haematologist would be helpful.

BIOCHEMISTRY

2

BIOCHEMISTRY

Urea and electrolyte profile

A urea and electrolyte profile (U&E) is the most commonly requested biochemical blood test. A U&E, in combination with a full blood picture (FBP), is performed for virtually all new hospital admissions. A U&E incorporates measures of electrolytes (sodium and potassium), along with renal function (urea and creatinine). A U&E is often used as a screening test in unwell patients, and frequently acts as a stimulus for further investigation.

Electrolyte abnormalities

Abnormalities in sodium and potassium occur when they are either too low (hyponatraemia – low sodium; hypokalaemia – low potassium) or too high (hypernatraemia – high sodium; hyperkalaemia – high potassium).

Hyponatraemia

This is defined as a sodium concentration less than 135 mmol/l. It is helpful to interpret a low sodium value in the context of a patient's fluid status. The causes may be narrowed down depending on whether the patient is fluid depleted, normovolaemic or fluid overloaded.

HYPONATRAEMIA IN THE FLUID-DEPLETED PATIENT

Diuretic therapy
Hypoadrenalism
Volume depletion
- vomiting and/or diarrhoea
- other large volume fluid losses (eg burns, fistula, haemorrhage)

HYPONATRAEMIA IN THE NORMOVOLAEMIC PATIENT

Syndrome of inappropriate antidiuretic hormone secretion (SIADH)
Hypothyroidism
Psychogenic polydipsia

For further details on SIADH, see page 122.

HYPONATRAEMIA IN THE FLUID-OVERLOADED PATIENT
Cardiac failure
Liver failure
Renal failure (especially nephrotic syndrome)
Hypoalbuminaemia

Hypernatraemia

This is defined as a sodium concentration of more than 145 mmol/l.

CAUSES OF HYPERNATRAEMIA
Diabetes insipidus
Poor water intake
Administration of excess sodium in intravenous fluids
Administration of drugs containing high concentrations of sodium

For further details on diabetes insipidus, see page 121.

Hypokalaemia

This is defined as a potassium concentration of less than 3.5 mmol/l.

CAUSES OF HYPOKALAEMIA
Drugs
• diuretic therapy
Intestinal losses
• excess vomiting (eg pyloric stenosis)
• profuse diarrhoea
• high stoma or fistula output
Renal tubular disease
• renal tubular acidosis or drug-induced tubular damage
Endocrine causes (eg Cushing's and Conn's syndromes)
Metabolic alkalosis

Hypokalaemia is associated with characteristic changes on the ECG. This is discussed on page 262.

Hyperkalaemia

This is defined as a potassium concentration of more than 4.5 mmol/l.

CAUSES OF HYPERKALAEMIA

Renal failure
Haemolysis of blood sample in transit (artefactual hyperkalaemia)
Drugs
- excess potassium supplementation
- potassium-sparing diuretics
- combination of drugs (eg angiotensin-converting enzyme (ACE) inhibitor and diuretic)
Rhabdomyolysis
Endocrine diseases (eg Addison's disease)
Diabetic ketoacidosis

Hyperkalaemia is associated with characteristic changes on the ECG. This is discussed on page 262.

DON'T FORGET

Hyperkalaemia is a medical emergency with levels of potassium of more than 6.5 mmol/l requiring immediate attention

Renal function

The presence of a normal urea and creatinine level is not synonymous with normal renal function. A thin elderly woman may have significant renal impairment despite her creatinine appearing within the 'normal' laboratory range. One must pay attention to the age, sex and muscle bulk of a patient when interpreting the significance of a creatinine level.

For accurate measurement of renal function, estimation of the glomerular filtration rate (GFR) is required.

DON'T FORGET

A normal GFR is considered to be approximately 100 ml/min per 1.73 m^2

Estimated GFR

Recently a method of calculating an estimated GFR (eGFR, in ml/min) on the basis of serum creatinine, age, sex and race has become widely recognised. It is calculated as shown in the boxes below.

ESTIMATED GFR

$eGFR = 186 \times (P_{Cr}/88.4)^{-1.154} \times A^{-0.203}$

where P_{Cr} is plasma creatinine concentration (µmol/l) and A is age in years

Correction factors for gender (0.742 female) and for race (1.210 black) are needed

---

Computer programs are available for assistance with the mathematics.

EXAMPLE CALCULATION

For a 62-year-old black female patient with a plasma creatinine of 150 µmol/l the eGFR would be calculated as:

$eGFR = 186 \times (150/88.4)^{-1.154} \times (62)^{-0.203} \times 0.742 \times 1.210 = 39.3$ (in ml/min)

Creatinine clearance

'Creatinine clearance' provides another useful indication of the GFR and can be measured in one of two ways.

Method 1

This requires a single blood creatinine value and a 24-h collection of urine.

$$CL_{Cr} = \frac{U_{Cr} \times \dot{U}}{P_{Cr}}$$

where CL_{Cr} is the creatinine clearance (ml/min), U_{Cr} is the concentration of creatinine in the urine (mmol/l), $\dot{U}$ is the urine flow rate (ml/min) and P_{Cr} is the concentration of creatinine in plasma (mmol/l)

Difficulties in this method of calculation arise for two reasons

1. The plasma creatinine is usually measured in μmol/l, not mmol/l as required by the formula.

2. Urine flow rate is usually measured in litres per 24 h, ie the amount of urine produced in one day (1440 min).

Hence a correction factor of 0.694 is required (1000/1440).

To account for this, use the following modified formula:

$$CL_{Cr} = \frac{U_{cr} \times V \times 0.694)}{B_{Cr}}$$

where V = 24 h urine volume (ml)
B_{Cr} = concentration creatinine in plasma (μmol/l)

EXAMPLE CALCULATION

For a patient with a plasma creatinine of 150 µmol/l, a 24-h urine volume of 2 l and a urinary creatinine concentration of 10 mmol/l, the creatinine clearance would be calculated as:

$$CL_{Cr} = \frac{10 \times 2000 \times 0.694}{150} = 92.5 \text{ (ml/min)}$$

Method 2

This method requires knowledge of the patient's age (A in years), weight (M in kg), sex and serum creatinine concentration (P_{Cr} in mg/dl).

$$CL_{Cr} = \frac{[(140 - A) \times M]}{72 \times P_{Cr}}$$

The formula generates an estimate of creatinine clearance for male patients. For females, the result of this calculation should be multiplied by 0.85.

Difficulties in this method of calculation arise because plasma creatinine is usually measured in µmol/l. To convert from µmol/l to mg/dl, divide by 88.4.

EXAMPLE CALCULATION

For a 66-year-old, 70-kg, female patient with a plasma creatinine of 150 µmol/l, the creatinine clearance would be calculated as:

$$CL_{Cr} = \frac{[(140 - 66) \times 70]}{(72 \times 150 \div 88.4)} = 42.4 \text{ ml/min}$$

Serum urea

The level of urea is reflective of both its production and elimination. Poor dietary intake can lead to a low urea level. Elevations in urea levels occur in renal failure, but are also commonly seen following a gastrointestinal bleed. Blood is effectively an excess protein load which is digested by the bowel.

Plasma osmolarity

Serum osmolarity can be calculated using the results of a U+E with the blood glucose level. Osmolarity is determined by the concentration of osmotically active particles of which sodium is the most influential. It is calculated as follows.

Plasma osmolarity = $2 \times (P_{Na} + P_K) + P_{Urea} + P_{Glucose}$
where P_{Na} is plasma sodium, P_K plasma potassium, P_{Urea} plasma urea and $P_{Glucose}$ is plasma glucose, all in mmol/l

Nutritional profile

A nutritional profile comprises measures of magnesium, calcium, phosphate and albumin. In patients with poor nutrition, all these nutrients may be deficient. Commonly deficiencies are seen in patients with poor oral diets (eg alcoholics, hunger strikers), or in patients with malabsorption. Further tests are available to provide blood levels of trace metals such as selenium.

Urine in acute renal failure

Acute renal failure is a common problem in clinical practice. The commonest cause of this is renal hypoperfusion. Urine is often analysed for electrolyte content in such patients to enable the differentiation of pre-renal uraemia from acute tubular necrosis. Patients with pre-renal uraemia would be expected to recover faster than those with acute tubular necrosis when appropriate therapy is initiated.

The key to correct interpretation of urinary electrolytes is understanding that in pre-renal uraemia, normal renal regulatory mechanisms remain intact and attempt to maintain homeostasis. The juxtaglomerular apparatus senses the reduction in renal blood flow and activates the renin–angiotensin–aldosterone system. The end-product, aldosterone, acts to promote sodium reabsorption in the distal convoluted tubule. This results in an increase in the circulating volume. Therefore, in pre-renal uraemia, the urinary sodium is low.

In acute tubular necrosis, the normal physiological mechanisms break down. Urinary sodium is therefore high.

It is difficult to interpret urinary sodium levels when a patient is taking a salt-wasting diuretic

The fractional sodium excretion (FE_{Na}) is sometimes measured in addition. This is simply a measure of the proportion of sodium that is filtered at the glomerulus that ends up in the urine. The FE_{Na} will therefore be low in pre-renal uraemia and high in acute tubular necrosis.

The following table summarises the differences.

	PRE-RENAL URAEMIA	ACUTE TUBULAR NECROSIS
Urinary sodium (mmol/l)	<20	>40
FE_{Na} (%)	<1	>1
Urine concentration	Concentrated	Relatively dilute

Case 11

A 76-year-old woman is admitted unwell with vomiting and is found to have a low blood pressure. She had recently been given diclofenac following a complaint of back pain. Her initial blood results included a U+E.

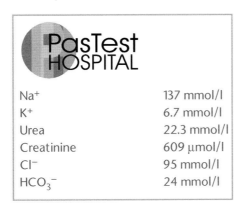

PasTest
HOSPITAL

Na^+	137 mmol/l
K^+	6.7 mmol/l
Urea	22.3 mmol/l
Creatinine	609 µmol/l
Cl^-	95 mmol/l
HCO_3^-	24 mmol/l

1. **What has happened to this patient?**

2. **What immediate treatment is indicated?**

Answer 11

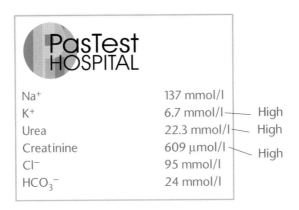

Na$^+$	137 mmol/l	
K$^+$	6.7 mmol/l	High
Urea	22.3 mmol/l	High
Creatinine	609 μmol/l	High
Cl$^-$	95 mmol/l	
HCO$_3^-$	24 mmol/l	

1. The urea and creatinine are both grossly elevated indicating that this patient has renal failure. Comparison with previous blood tests would indicate whether this is acute or chronic. As a consequence of the renal failure, serum potassium is dangerously elevated. The rising potassium is a reflection of the failing tubular function of the kidney. In this case it would appear that the use of a non-steroidal anti-inflammatory drug (diclofenac) and vomiting are the causes of an acute deterioration in renal function.

2. Hyperkalaemia can cause fatal dysrhythmias, including cardiac arrest. This requires immediate treatment. Conventional treatment employs insulin and dextrose. Insulin drives potassium into the cells, while glucose prevents hypoglycaemia. Calcium gluconate should be given to stabilise the myocardium.

   The ultimate treatment is to identify the cause of the renal failure and support the kidneys until function is restored.

Case 12

A 49-year-old missionary is brought to your hospital by his wife. He has been vomiting for the past 24 h. He is now very weak. He last ate 2 days previously and has struggled to keep down any liquids since. On examination his mouth is dry, his abdomen is generally uncomfortable and he has reduced skin turgor. After taking his routine blood tests, a 0.9% saline drip is erected before any results are checked. A short time later the following result is available.

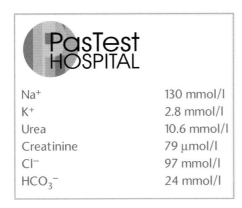

Na^+	130 mmol/l
K^+	2.8 mmol/l
Urea	10.6 mmol/l
Creatinine	79 μmol/l
Cl^-	97 mmol/l
HCO_3^-	24 mmol/l

1.   Outline the abnormalities on this blood result.

After noting the above results, his IV fluid prescription is changed to 1 litre of 0.9% saline containing 40 mmol/l of potassium chloride, to be infused over 6 h.

Two hours later, his U&E is repeated, and is shown below.

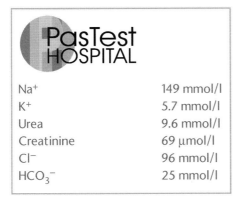

Na^+	149 mmol/l
K^+	5.7 mmol/l
Urea	9.6 mmol/l
Creatinine	69 μmol/l
Cl^-	96 mmol/l
HCO_3^-	25 mmol/l

The ward doctor is concerned, and a further sample is taken.

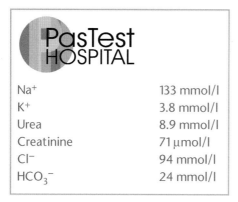

PasTest
HOSPITAL

Na^+	133 mmol/l
K^+	3.8 mmol/l
Urea	8.9 mmol/l
Creatinine	71 µmol/l
Cl^-	94 mmol/l
HCO_3^-	24 mmol/l

2. **How would you account for the discrepancy between these two blood tests?**

Answer 12

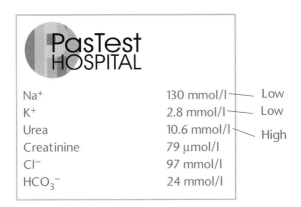

PasTest
HOSPITAL

Na$^+$	130 mmol/l	Low
K$^+$	2.8 mmol/l	Low
Urea	10.6 mmol/l	High
Creatinine	79 µmol/l	
Cl$^-$	97 mmol/l	
HCO$_3$$^-$	24 mmol/l	

1. Three abnormalities can be seen in the results above:

- Low sodium (hyponatraemia)

- Low potassium (hypokalaemia)

- High urea (uraemia).

The low sodium and low potassium are a consequence of a prolonged period of vomiting combined with very limited oral intake. There has been a substantial loss of electrolytes without any means of replacement until admission to hospital. The patient is clinically dehydrated and the raised urea is a reflection of this.

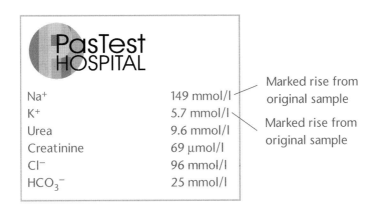

PasTest
HOSPITAL

Na$^+$	149 mmol/l	Marked rise from original sample
K$^+$	5.7 mmol/l	
Urea	9.6 mmol/l	Marked rise from original sample
Creatinine	69 µmol/l	
Cl$^-$	96 mmol/l	
HCO$_3$$^-$	25 mmol/l	

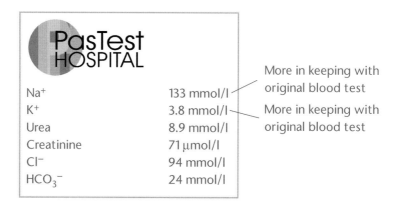

PasTest
HOSPITAL

Na⁺	133 mmol/l	More in keeping with original blood test
K⁺	3.8 mmol/l	More in keeping with original blood test
Urea	8.9 mmol/l	
Creatinine	71 µmol/l	
Cl⁻	94 mmol/l	
HCO₃⁻	24 mmol/l	

2. Looking at the first repeat blood test, the sodium and potassium levels have both risen from the time of admission a few hours previously. There has been a dramatic change in electrolyte levels. The second repeat sample is very different again.

The explanation for these findings is that the first repeat blood sample has been taken from the arm into which fluid is being infused. This is an erroneous sample.

The second repeat sample comes from a 'non-drip' arm, and shows the true state of affairs, ie slowly improving electrolytes from the time of admission.

Case 13

A 34-year-old man is admitted with epigastric discomfort and a single episode of vomiting following a week-long binge of alcohol. His vital signs are within the normal range. Blood tests were taken at the time of admission.

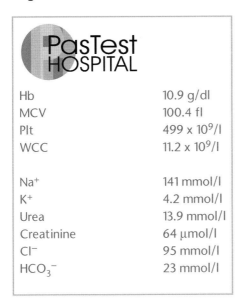

PasTest HOSPITAL	
Hb	10.9 g/dl
MCV	100.4 fl
Plt	499 x 10^9/l
WCC	11.2 x 10^9/l
Na$^+$	141 mmol/l
K$^+$	4.2 mmol/l
Urea	13.9 mmol/l
Creatinine	64 µmol/l
Cl$^-$	95 mmol/l
HCO$_3^-$	23 mmol/l

Explain the elevated urea in the context of the other haematological results.

Answer 13

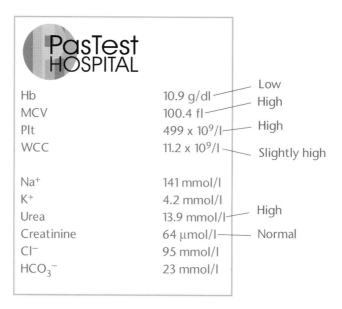

PasTest
HOSPITAL

Hb	10.9 g/dl	Low High
MCV	100.4 fl	High
Plt	499 x 10⁹/l	High
WCC	11.2 x 10⁹/l	Slightly high
Na⁺	141 mmol/l	
K⁺	4.2 mmol/l	
Urea	13.9 mmol/l	High
Creatinine	64 μmol/l	Normal
Cl⁻	95 mmol/l	
HCO₃⁻	23 mmol/l	

This man's U&E reveals an elevated urea. His creatinine is normal and his clinical history does not suggest dehydration. His full blood count reveals information which helps in interpreting the significance of the elevated urea. His haemoglobin, MCV, white cell count and platelets are all abnormal. The raised MCV most likely represents chronic alcohol use.

During gastrointestinal bleeding, an increase in urea may occur. This is because urea is a breakdown product of digested blood. Similarly during an active bleed, a rise in the white cell count and platelet count may occur.

The combination of the following is suggestive of gastrointestinal bleeding:

- raised urea (with normal creatinine)
- low haemoglobin
- raised white cell count (in the absence of infection)
- raised platelets.

Case 14

A 46-year-old diplomat is transferred to your care following medical evacuation from Nigeria. In his transfer correspondence it indicates that he has developed renal impairment which as yet has not been investigated in depth.

His U&E is shown, along with a 24-h urine collection for creatinine clearance.

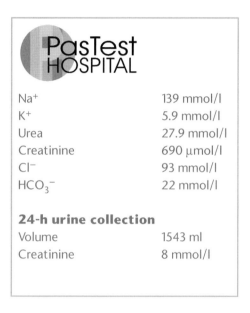

PasTest HOSPITAL

Na$^+$	139 mmol/l
K$^+$	5.9 mmol/l
Urea	27.9 mmol/l
Creatinine	690 µmol/l
Cl$^-$	93 mmol/l
HCO$_3^-$	22 mmol/l

24-h urine collection

Volume	1543 ml
Creatinine	8 mmol/l

Calculate his creatinine clearance.

Answer 14

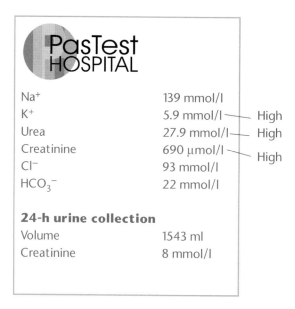

PasTest HOSPITAL

Na$^+$	139 mmol/l
K$^+$	5.9 mmol/l —— High
Urea	27.9 mmol/l —— High
Creatinine	690 µmol/l —— High
Cl$^-$	93 mmol/l
HCO$_3^-$	22 mmol/l

24-h urine collection

Volume	1543 ml
Creatinine	8 mmol/l

Creatinine clearance can be calculated using the following equation:

$$CL_{Cr} = \frac{U_{Cr} \times V \times 0.694}{B_{Cr}}$$

where V_{Cr} is the concentration of creatinine in urine (in mmol/l), V is the 24-h urine volume (in ml) and B_{Cr} is plasma creatinine in µmol/l

In this case:

$$CL_{Cr} = \frac{8 \times 1543 \times 0.694}{690} = 12.4 \text{ ml/min}$$

The creatinine clearance is 12.4 ml/min. Bearing in mind that the normal creatinine clearance is approximately 100 ml/min, it is clear that this man has significant renal impairment.

Case 15

A 22-year-old university student is trapped in her house during a fire and when rescued by firefighters has developed substantial burns to the arms and chest. She is admitted to the Burns Unit. A U&E on her third day is shown.

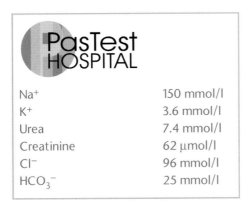

PasTest
HOSPITAL

Na^+	150 mmol/l
K^+	3.6 mmol/l
Urea	7.4 mmol/l
Creatinine	62 µmol/l
Cl^-	96 mmol/l
HCO_3^-	25 mmol/l

What is the main biochemical problem and name some of its causes?

Answer 15

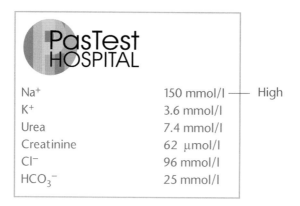

PasTest
HOSPITAL

Na$^+$	150 mmol/l	High
K$^+$	3.6 mmol/l	
Urea	7.4 mmol/l	
Creatinine	62 μmol/l	
Cl$^-$	96 mmol/l	
HCO$_3$$^-$	25 mmol/l	

Hypernatraemia is present. Other components of the U&E are normal. The commonest cause for this observation in hospital medicine is excessive use of 0.9% saline in those patients receiving IV fluids. This is one reason why IV fluid prescribing should be considered carefully and regular U&E samples checked. This is especially important in patients with excessive fluid losses, such as patients with burns. In this patient, substantial fluid loss from her burns has led to a water deficit. Consequentially, the sodium concentration has risen.

Other causes of hypernatraemia are listed on page 44.

Case 16

A 39-year-old man with a history of Crohn's disease and previous extensive small bowel resection is admitted with anorexia and weight loss. His GP is very concerned that he now weighs only 39 kg and has not been able to tolerate much in the way of oral foods for several months. In hospital, attempts were made to start naso-gastric feeding, but it could not be tolerated. Total parenteral nutrition (TPN) was therefore commenced. The following table shows his U&E and nutritional profile over several days following commencement of parenteral feeding.

PasTest HOSPITAL

Date	14/02	15/02	16/02	17/02
Na^+ (mmol/l)	135	135	134	136
K^+ (mmol/l)	3.3	3.4	3.4	3.7
Urea (mmol/l)	2.1	2.2	2.2	2.3
Creatinine (μmol/l)	44	49	47	45
Cl^- (mmol/l)	94	94	93	93
HCO_3^- (mmol/l)	23	22	23	23
Mg^{2+} (mmol/l)	0.39	0.37	0.38	0.51
PO_4^{3-} (mmol/l)	0.70	0.61	0.41	0.40
Total Ca^{2+} (mmol/l)	2.32	2.05	2.12	2.22
Albumin (g/l)	33	32	33	32

Comment on these results.

Answer 16

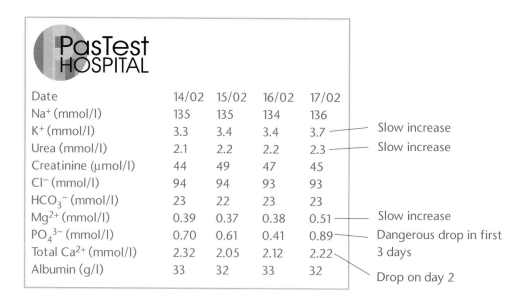

Date	14/02	15/02	16/02	17/02	
Na^+ (mmol/l)	135	135	134	136	
K^+ (mmol/l)	3.3	3.4	3.4	3.7	Slow increase
Urea (mmol/l)	2.1	2.2	2.2	2.3	Slow increase
Creatinine (µmol/l)	44	49	47	45	
Cl^- (mmol/l)	94	94	93	93	
HCO_3^- (mmol/l)	23	22	23	23	
Mg^{2+} (mmol/l)	0.39	0.37	0.38	0.51	Slow increase
PO_4^{3-} (mmol/l)	0.70	0.61	0.41	0.89	Dangerous drop in first
Total Ca^{2+} (mmol/l)	2.32	2.05	2.12	2.22	3 days
Albumin (g/l)	33	32	33	32	Drop on day 2

This scenario illustrates the issue of re-feeding in those patients who have been nutritionally depleted for some time. When feeding is commenced, a rapid and precipitous drop often occurs, in particular, phosphate levels.

Bone profile

In health, bone undergoes a continuous process of remodelling by osteoclasts and osteoblasts. A bone profile is a batch of biochemical blood tests grouped together as they are all relevant to bone disease. It comprises calcium, phosphate and alkaline phosphatase (ALP). Albumin is also included for reasons detailed below. Metabolic bone diseases are associated with characteristic abnormalities on the bone profile. More specialised analyses, for example parathyroid hormone (PTH) or vitamin D levels, can be carried out when clinically relevant.

COMPONENTS OF A BONE PROFILE
Calcium
Phosphate
Alkaline phosphatase
Albumin

Calcium homeostasis is under hormonal control with PTH being a key regulator. When calcium is low, PTH is released. This acts to raise serum calcium levels by:

- increasing calcium resorption from bone

- increasing renal calcium reabsorption

- increasing renal excretion of phosphate

- indirectly increasing absorption of calcium from the gut via effects on vitamin D.

Major metabolic bone diseases

The major bone diseases that a student might be expected to identify from a bone profile are listed in the box below.

MAJOR BONE DISEASES	
Osteoporosis	Bony metastases
Osteomalacia	Hyperparathyroidism
Paget's disease	

Typical patterns of results are shown in the following box.

BONE DISEASES	CALCIUM	PHOSPHATE	ALP
Osteoporosis	N	N	N
Osteomalacia	N/↓	↓	↑
Paget's disease	N	N	↑
Bony metastases	↑/N	N/↑	↑
Primary hyperparathyroidism	↑	↓	↑
Secondary hyperparathyroidism	N	↑	↑
Tertiary hyperparathyroidism	↑	↓	↑

DON'T FORGET

The bone profile is normal in osteoporosis

Corrected calcium

It is important to appreciate that a high proportion of calcium is bound to protein (albumin). However, it is the unbound calcium that is most important physiologically. For this reason when protein (albumin) is low the total calcium level may be misleading and a correction calculation needs to be made. The 'corrected calcium' level refers to the calcium level corrected for the fact that the albumin is abnormal. Corrected calcium can be calculated as follows:

$$P_{Ca}C = P_{Ca} + \frac{(0.1\,(40-\text{Alb (g/l)})}{4}$$

where $P_{Ca}C$ (in mmol/l) is the corrected calcium level, P_{Ca} (in mmol/l) is the calcium level and Alb is the albumin concentration (g/l).

EXAMPLE CALCULATION

If: Calcium = 1.92 mmol/l
Albumin = 20 g/l $P_{Ca}C$ (mmol/l) = 1.92 + $\dfrac{[0.1 \times (40-20)]}{4}$ = 2.42 mmol/l

Case 17

A 72-year-old former engine driver attends his GP complaining of generalised aches and pains. During the consultation you have to speak loudly to be understood. As part of your investigations you request a bone profile. Liver function tests were normal.

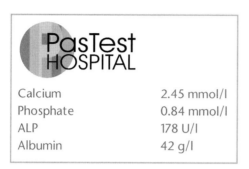

PasTest HOSPITAL	
Calcium	2.45 mmol/l
Phosphate	0.84 mmol/l
ALP	178 U/l
Albumin	42 g/l

On the basis of this test he received a course of treatment for several months. Following treatment his bone profile is repeated and is as follows.

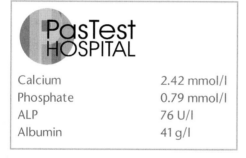

PasTest HOSPITAL	
Calcium	2.42 mmol/l
Phosphate	0.79 mmol/l
ALP	76 U/l
Albumin	41 g/l

1. **What bone disease does this patient have?**

2. **What treatment is he likely to have received to explain the change in his bone profile?**

Answer 17

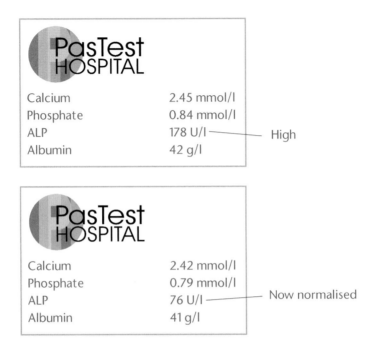

PasTest HOSPITAL

Calcium	2.45 mmol/l
Phosphate	0.84 mmol/l
ALP	178 U/l —— High
Albumin	42 g/l

PasTest HOSPITAL

Calcium	2.42 mmol/l
Phosphate	0.79 mmol/l
ALP	76 U/l —— Now normalised
Albumin	41 g/l

1. This elderly man has Paget's disease of the bone. He has an isolated ALP rise, in the absence of any liver disease. An ALP rise can occur for various reasons, including primary sclerosing cholangitis and bony metastases. However, in the context of this patient's symptoms, with deafness, Paget's disease is most likely.

2. The repeat bone profile demonstrates lowering of the ALP after successful treatment. He is likely to have received intravenous bisphosphonate therapy. Note that the majority of patients with Paget's disease are asymptomatic and the disease is often diagnosed incidentally when tests are requested for other reasons.

Case 18

A 69-year-old retired nurse complains of generalised aches and pains for the past 5 weeks, sometimes preventing her from sleeping at night. Her past medical history includes hypothyroidism, hypertension and a mastectomy 14 years ago for breast carcinoma. She is a very active member of the Women's Institute and feels less able to complete her daily tasks of late.

Blood tests included a bone profile. Liver function tests were normal.

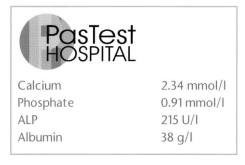

Calcium	2.34 mmol/l
Phosphate	0.91 mmol/l
ALP	215 U/l
Albumin	38 g/l

Describe the findings on the bone profile and give an explanation.

Answer 18

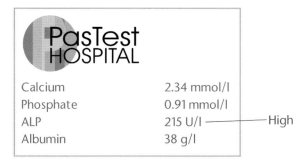

Calcium	2.34 mmol/l
Phosphate	0.91 mmol/l
ALP	215 U/l ——————High
Albumin	38 g/l

The ALP is significantly raised. The rest of the bone profile is normal. ALP may be high in a number of conditions. It is important to exclude liver disease, but we are told here that the rest of her liver function tests were normal.

Bearing in mind the clinical history, a particular concern in this woman would be bony metastases from breast carcinoma. This can occur a considerable time after treatment of the primary tumour. The calcium may be normal or elevated in the presence of bony metastases.

Case 19

A 45-year-old teacher has been complaining of aches and pains for several months. Her colleagues have said that she has not been herself recently, appearing 'under the weather' and sad. She is still menstruating regularly. Among the blood tests requested by her GP was a bone profile.

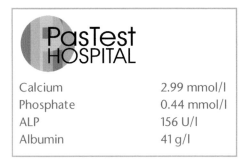

PasTest HOSPITAL	
Calcium	2.99 mmol/l
Phosphate	0.44 mmol/l
ALP	156 U/l
Albumin	41 g/l

A further blood test, of great importance in diagnosis, was sent the following day.

1. **What is the additional test likely to be?**

2. **What is the likely diagnosis?**

Answer 19

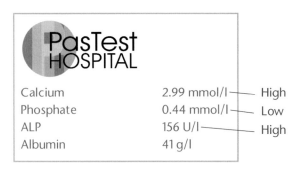

PasTest HOSPITAL		
Calcium	2.99 mmol/l—	High
Phosphate	0.44 mmol/l—	Low
ALP	156 U/l—	High
Albumin	41 g/l	

1. The additional test is for parathyroid hormone (PTH).

2. These findings are in keeping with primary hyperparathyroidism.

The excess PTH, most likely from a parathyroid adenoma, is causing excess bone resorption resulting in a high calcium and ALP. Constitutional symptoms include bony aches, low mood and constipation, which can arise due to the hypercalcaemia. Hence the patient with hyperparathyroidism can have problems with 'bones, stones, moans and abdominal groans'.

Note that in primary hyperparathyroidism PTH is generally raised. However, a normal PTH level is also abnormal in a patient with hypercalcaemia and may be indicative of hyperparathyroidism. This is because PTH should normally be suppressed by negative feedback in the setting of hypercalcaemia.

Case 20

A 46-year-old office clerk attends a private health clinic complaining of aches in his bones and tenderness over his muscles. This has been troubling him for some time and he is no longer able to walk to work. He has suffered from coeliac disease for many years, but by his own confession finds it hard at times to stick to his gluten-free diet. A 'screen' of tests is taken, some of which are shown below.

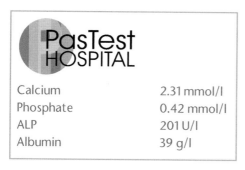

PasTest HOSPITAL	
Calcium	2.31 mmol/l
Phosphate	0.42 mmol/l
ALP	201 U/l
Albumin	39 g/l

What is the likely diagnosis?

Answer 20

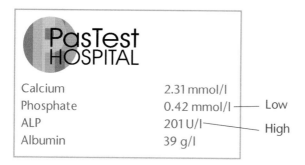

PasTest HOSPITAL		
Calcium	2.31 mmol/l	
Phosphate	0.42 mmol/l	— Low
ALP	201 U/l	— High
Albumin	39 g/l	

These findings are in keeping with a diagnosis of osteomalacia. Osteomalacia is a metabolic bone disease in which there is a lack of calcium or phosphate (or both) for mineralisation of newly formed osteoid. As a result, bone is 'soft' and unable to withstand the stresses and forces of normal bone. Parathyroid hormone would need to be checked if there was any diagnostic doubt.

It is likely that this patient's coeliac disease is contributing to the development of osteomalacia through malabsorption of calcium.

Case 21

A 55-year-old woman is admitted with a fractured neck of femur after a minor trip in the car park of her local supermarket. Looking back through her old records, the admitting doctor notices the following bone profile taken 2 weeks previously.

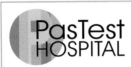

Calcium	2.31 mmol/l
Phosphate	0.87 mmol/l
ALP	69 U/l
Albumin	39 g/l

What bone disease might you suspect?

Answer 21

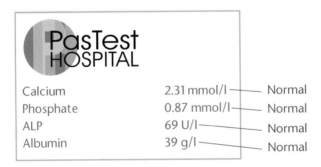

Calcium	2.31 mmol/l	Normal
Phosphate	0.87 mmol/l	Normal
ALP	69 U/l	Normal
Albumin	39 g/l	Normal

You should suspect osteoporosis given the history of fracture after minimal trauma, and a previously normal bone profile. Osteoporosis is the commonest form of metabolic bone disease. It is predominantly found in postmenopausal women and is considered a silent disease. First presentation is often with a low trauma fracture as in this clinical scenario.

Diagnosis of osteoporosis is usually made using dual energy X-ray absorptiometry (DEXA).

Liver function tests

Liver function tests (LFTs) comprise six measurements: bilirubin, aspartate transaminase (AST), alanine aminotransferase (ALT), alkaline phosphatase (ALP), gamma-glutamyl transpeptidase (GGT) and albumin. Prothrombin time (PTT) which is part of a coagulation screen is an important addition (see page 18).

COMPONENTS OF LIVER FUNCTION TESTS
Bilirubin
Aspartate transaminase
Alanine aminotransferase
Alkaline phosphatase
Gamma-glutamyl transpeptidase
Albumin

Note that AST and ALP are not tests specific to the liver. AST is also released when muscle (including cardiac muscle) is damaged. ALP is raised in a number of bone diseases, hence its presence in a bone profile.

If these basic LFTs are abnormal, further specific tests may be performed to establish an underlying cause.

TEST	DISEASE	EXPECTED RESULT
Autoantibody screen	Autoimmune hepatitis	Anti-nuclear Anti-smooth muscle Anti-liver/kidney microsomal-I
	Primary biliary cirrhosis	Anti-mitochondrial
Iron profile	Haemochromatosis	High iron and ferritin Low TIBC
Copper studies	Wilson's disease	Low caeruloplasmin
Viral hepatitis 'screen'	Hepatitis	Positive antigen presence

Broadly speaking, disturbances of liver function may be classified into three patterns:

- Hepatitic (parenchymal)
- Obstructive
- Mixed.

These patterns assist in narrowing the differential diagnosis of altered liver function. An understanding of the different causes allows an appropriate sequence of investigation.

When hepatocellular damage occurs, hepatocytes 'spill out' transaminases (AST and ALT). A rise in these indices alone may be termed a 'transaminitis'.

When there is obstruction to the outflow of bile from the liver, an obstructive pattern (elevated ALP and GGT) will be seen. The bilirubin level would also be expected to be high.

Bilirubin is conjugated in the liver with the attachment of a glucuronide group. This measured bilirubin may be conjugated (direct bilirubin) or unconjugated (indirect bilirubin). Total bilirubin is the sum of both types.

Confusion sometimes arises in obstructive liver disease when the AST and ALT are also elevated. This occurs because of back pressure on the liver. In such instances the elevation of ALP and GGT will be out of proportion to that of the transaminases.

CAUSES OF HEPATITIC LFTs

- Viral hepatitis
- Autoimmune hepatitis
- Drugs and toxins
- Alcohol
- Metabolic disorders (eg Wilson's disease)
- Fatty liver
- Malignancy (both primary and metastatic)
- Congestive cardiac failure

CAUSES OF OBSTRUCTIVE LFTs

Obstruction in the bile duct lumen
- Bile duct gallstone

An abnormal bile duct wall
- Bile duct stricture
- Cholangiocarcinoma

Compression of the bile duct by an extrinsic lesion
- Pancreatic carcinoma
- Nodes at the porta hepatis
- Ampullary carcinoma

One of the functions of the liver is protein synthesis. In a failing liver, synthetic function is often affected. This will manifest as low albumin levels and a raised prothrombin time (since the liver manufactures clotting factors).

Case 22

A 68-year-old woman was admitted with itch, lethargy and discoloration of the skin over the past month. On examination she is icteric and cachexic. There are no stigmata of chronic liver disease. Nursing staff indicate that there is discoloration of her urine.

Her admission bloods include LFTs.

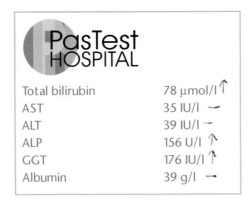

PasTest
HOSPITAL

Total bilirubin	78 μmol/l ↑
AST	35 IU/l →
ALT	39 IU/l →
ALP	156 U/l ↑
GGT	176 IU/l ↑
Albumin	39 g/l →

1. **Outline the abnormalities seen on the liver function tests.**

2. **What would be your next choice of investigation?**

3. **What are the potential causes of these results?**

Answer 22

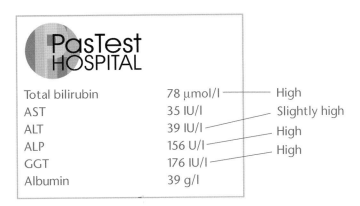

PasTest HOSPITAL		
Total bilirubin	78 µmol/l	High
AST	35 IU/l	Slightly high
ALT	39 IU/l	High
ALP	156 U/l	High
GGT	176 IU/l	
Albumin	39 g/l	

1. The LFTs show an elevated bilirubin with obstructive LFTs.

2. An ultrasound scan of the abdomen is the next most important investigation. This will confirm the presence of obstruction and may identify the underlying cause. This can then act as a guide for further investigations.

3. The causes of obstructive jaundice are listed on page 75.

Case 23

A 47-year-old woman is referred to the regional hepatology outpatient clinic by her GP. She attended her GP on several occasions complaining of tiredness, low mood, altered bowel habit and more recently of itch. On examination a 4-cm smooth hepatomegaly is noted, with xanthelasmata around her eyes.

The referral letter contains the following LFTs:

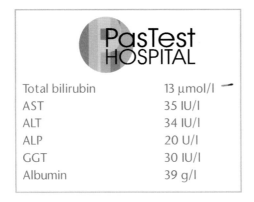

PasTest HOSPITAL	
Total bilirubin	13 µmol/l
AST	35 IU/l
ALT	34 IU/l
ALP	20 U/l
GGT	30 IU/l
Albumin	39 g/l

A blood test taken at the clinic revealed the following:

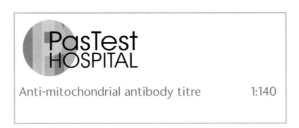

PasTest HOSPITAL	
Anti-mitochondrial antibody titre	1:140

1. **Interpret these results.**

2. **Suggest a further investigation.**

Answer 23

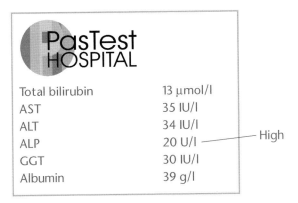

Total bilirubin	13 µmol/l
AST	35 IU/l
ALT	34 IU/l
ALP	20 U/l ——— High
GGT	30 IU/l
Albumin	39 g/l

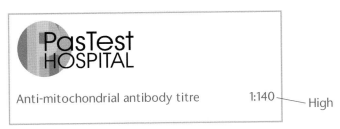

Anti-mitochondrial antibody titre	1:140 —— High

1. The only abnormality on the liver biochemistry is a raised ALP. ALP may be raised in bone as well as liver disease (see page 65). An isolated ALP rise may be seen in both primary sclerosing cholangitis (PSC) and early primary biliary cirrhosis (PBC). The normal albumin suggests that the synthetic function of the liver remains intact. The immunological tests are the diagnostic key in this case. A substantially raised anti-mitochondrial antibody (AMA) is observed. Ninety-five per cent of patients with PBC will have a positive antibody for AMA-M2. In PSC the presence of autoantibodies is uncommon.

2. The most useful investigation to confirm and assess the extent of disease would be a liver biopsy.

Case 24

A 34-year-old labourer is admitted with right upper quadrant discomfort, fever and sweats. He returned from a project overseas 3 weeks earlier. On examination he is tender to palpitation over the right hypochondrium making complete examination difficult. A spiking fever pattern is seen on his observation chart. His LFTs are as follows.

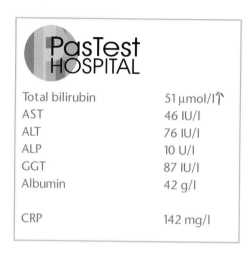

Total bilirubin	51 μmol/l↑
AST	46 IU/l
ALT	76 IU/l
ALP	10 U/l
GGT	87 IU/l
Albumin	42 g/l
CRP	142 mg/l

1. **What investigation does this patient need as soon as possible based on his clinical history and blood tests?**

2. **What is the likely diagnosis?**

Answer 24

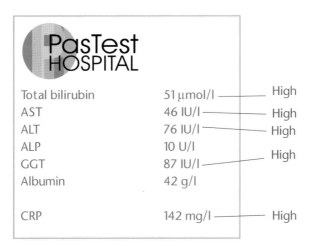

1. The bilirubin and transaminases are raised. The CRP is highly elevated. He requires an ultrasound scan of the abdomen to investigate an infective cause for his symptoms.

2. A liver abscess or cholangitis are potential causes.

Case 25

A 37-year-old manual worker is admitted with generalised abdominal discomfort, vomiting and shakiness. On examination there is a 4-cm mildly tender hepatomegaly. He is sweaty to the touch. Some blood tests are requested.

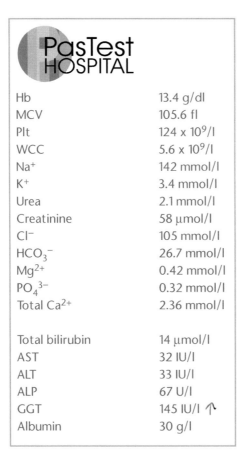

PasTest HOSPITAL

Hb	13.4 g/dl
MCV	105.6 fl
Plt	124 x 10^9/l
WCC	5.6 x 10^9/l
Na^+	142 mmol/l
K^+	3.4 mmol/l
Urea	2.1 mmol/l
Creatinine	58 µmol/l
Cl^-	105 mmol/l
HCO_3^-	26.7 mmol/l
Mg^{2+}	0.42 mmol/l
PO_4^{3-}	0.32 mmol/l
Total Ca^{2+}	2.36 mmol/l
Total bilirubin	14 µmol/l
AST	32 IU/l
ALT	33 IU/l
ALP	67 U/l
GGT	145 IU/l ↑
Albumin	30 g/l

1. **Outline the abnormalities on this set of blood results.**

2. **Explain the likely cause of the LFT abnormalities given the abnormalities in the other results.**

Answer 25

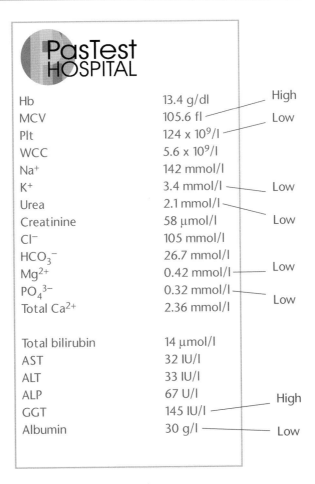

PasTest
HOSPITAL

Hb	13.4 g/dl	High
MCV	105.6 fl	Low
Plt	124 x 10^9/l	
WCC	5.6 x 10^9/l	
Na$^+$	142 mmol/l	
K$^+$	3.4 mmol/l	Low
Urea	2.1 mmol/l	
Creatinine	58 µmol/l	Low
Cl$^-$	105 mmol/l	
HCO$_3$$^-$	26.7 mmol/l	
Mg^{2+}	0.42 mmol/l	Low
PO$_4$$^{3-}$	0.32 mmol/l	
Total Ca^{2+}	2.36 mmol/l	Low
Total bilirubin	14 µmol/l	
AST	32 IU/l	
ALT	33 IU/l	
ALP	67 U/l	
GGT	145 IU/l	High
Albumin	30 g/l	Low

1. The abnormalities seen include:

   - a raised MCV, with a borderline low platelet count

   - low values for urea, potassium, magnesium and, in particular, phosphate

   - a raised GGT

   - a low albumin.

2. The findings on these simple blood tests are classic for an individual who has consumed large quantities of alcohol for a significant time period.

Case 26

A 44-year-old woman with primary biliary cirrhosis has been attending hepatology outpatients for many years. Over the past 18 months she has been feeling less well in herself and her frequency of attendance for review has increased at the insistence of her physician. On examination she is jaundiced and her abdomen is mildly distended with a 3-cm hepatomegaly.

Her recent blood results are shown.

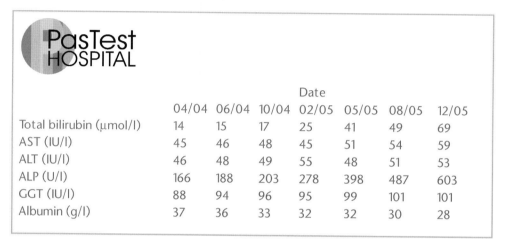

PasTest HOSPITAL

				Date			
	04/04	06/04	10/04	02/05	05/05	08/05	12/05
Total bilirubin (μmol/l)	14	15	17	25	41	49	69
AST (IU/l)	45	46	48	45	51	54	59
ALT (IU/l)	46	48	49	55	48	51	53
ALP (U/l)	166	188	203	278	398	487	603
GGT (IU/l)	88	94	96	95	99	101	101
Albumin (g/l)	37	36	33	32	32	30	28

Give a summary of the findings.

Answer 26

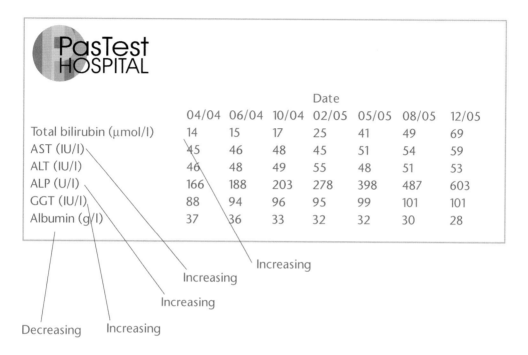

The course of primary biliary cirrhosis is variable. Patients may live with stable LFTs for a number of years. Decompensation may occur at any time with deterioration in the liver's synthetic ability indicating a failure of liver function.

The chart shows LFTs over a period of 20 months. Initially only a moderately elevated ALP is seen in April 2004. Over the ensuing months the ALP continues to rise, and with this the albumin falls reaching a low of 28 g/l in December 2005.

The prothrombin time should also be checked. One would expect it to be raised indicating impaired production of clotting factors by the failing liver.

Case 27

A 32-year-old man is recalled by his occupational health department following a recent 'medical' prior to transfer to an overseas operation within the company. He is teetotal. He cannot understand what all the fuss is about as he feels fine.

The blood results of concern are shown.

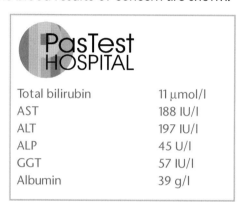

1. **What pattern of LFTs is demonstrated?**

2. **What further blood tests may help in coming to a diagnosis?**

Answer 27

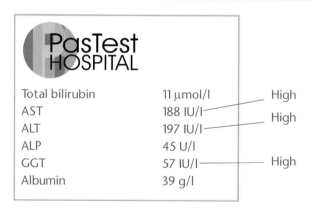

1. This patient has a parenchymal LFT derangement. Both the ALT and AST are markedly elevated.

2. The following blood tests should be performed to search for a cause of the abnormality: autoantibody screen, immunoglobins, renal function, iron profile, copper studies and viral hepatitis testing.

This patient had hepatitis C. Not infrequently hepatitis C is diagnosed incidentally when LFTs are checked for some other reason.

Cardiac enzymes

Cardiac enzymes are most commonly used to assist in the diagnosis of myocardial infarction and other acute coronary syndromes. Traditionally, a range of blood tests has been analysed in the search for evidence of cardiac damage. These test enzymes vary in the time taken for them to peak and to be cleared from the blood after a cardiac event. Differences in the tests are shown in the table below.

TEST	TIME TO PEAK (H)	DURATION OF ELEVATED BLOOD LEVEL AFTER CARDIAC EVENT
Creatine kinase (CK)	24	48
AST	30	60
Lactate dehydrogenase (LDH)	72	240

Creatine kinase is also released from damaged skeletal muscle. Its level will therefore rise in several instances other than myocardial damage, such as trauma, polymyositis/dermatomyositis (when muscle is inflamed) and rhabdomyolysis (when muscle breaks down). To aid differentiation between these conditions, isoenzymes (different types) of CK can be measured. The isoenzyme released mainly from cardiac muscle is called CK-MB, and a high level of this enzyme should raise suspicions of cardiac damage.

Increasingly, however, reliance is being placed on measures of serum troponins (types I or T) when testing for myocardial damage. These proteins are normally involved in cardiac muscle cell contraction, and are released systemically when cardiac muscle cells are damaged. Troponin measurement is the most specific test available for the assessment of myocardial damage. Troponins may be elevated after 2 h, and stay elevated for up to 7 days. Levels are generally measured 12 h after the onset of symptoms. Elevated troponin levels can be found in conditions other than myocardial infarction, as shown in the box below.

CAUSES OF RAISED TROPONIN	
• Myocardial infarction	• Renal failure
• Heart failure	• Severe sepsis
• Myocarditis	• Supraventricular tachycardia
• Pulmonary embolism	

C-reactive protein

C-reactive protein (CRP) is a protein produced in the liver. It is an acute phase reactant, being raised in inflammation and infection. It is often thought of in a similar manner to the erythrocyte sedimentation rate (ESR) (see page 15). The CRP and ESR are together termed inflammatory markers. There are a few recognised conditions in which the ESR is raised, but the CRP is normal.

CAUSES OF A RAISED ESR WITH A NORMAL CRP
SLE
Multiple myeloma

The level of the CRP is not necessarily reflective of the severity of a disease process.

Urate (uric acid)

Urate is produced during the metabolism of purines, and is excreted by the kidneys. High levels in the blood (hyperuricaemia) can occur through two mechanisms:

- increased purine consumption or uric acid production
- impaired excretion of uric acid.

A modest amount of the body's purines are ingested in food and drink. A patient with a raised urate level may be asymptomatic or may be troubled with gout. It is common practice to measure serum urate levels in any patient with an acute monoarthritis. High levels of urate may support a diagnosis of gout. However, urate levels may be normal during an acute attack of gout.

DON'T FORGET

Urate levels may be normal during an acute attack of gout

Tumour markers

Tumour markers are a selection of blood tests that are commonly elevated in patients with neoplastic disease. Most tumour markers are characteristically associated with a particular type of cancer, as shown in the table.

TUMOUR MARKER	ASSOCIATED TUMOURS
α Fetoprotein (α-FP)	Hepatocellular carcinoma; testicular teratoma
Human chorionic gonadotrophin (β-hCG)	Testicular teratoma and seminoma
Prostate-specific antigen (PSA)	Prostate
CA-125	Ovarian
CA-19-9	Pancreatic
Carcinoembryonic antigen (CEA)	Colorectal

However, with the exception of α-FP, β-HCG and PSA, tumour markers are fairly non-specific, and several markers may be elevated with one underlying cancer. Tumour markers should therefore be requested only when the significance of a positive result can be usefully interpreted.

Tumour markers have two chief roles in clinical practice. First, specific markers such as PSA can be used in making a diagnosis. Second, serial measures of tumour markers can be used to monitor disease progress and response to treatment.

DON'T FORGET

Tumour markers are isolated blood tests – interpret them in the context of clinical features and all allied investigations

Sweat testing

Cystic fibrosis results from a mutation in the gene that encodes the cystic fibrosis transmembrane conductance regulator (CFTR). CFTR is responsible for chloride ion transport across epithelial cells, and abnormalities in its structure result in viscous secretions particularly in the lung and pancreas.

Abnormal sweat gland function leads to high concentrations of sodium and chloride in the sweat. Indeed, excessively salty tasting sweat was noted to be a clinical feature of cystic fibrosis long before the genetics were fully understood. This feature underlies the diagnostic test for cystic fibrosis – the sweat test.

In this test, sweating is stimulated, and sweat collected for analysis. Sufficient sweat (100 mg) must be collected for the test to be reliable. The test is positive if more than 60 mmol/l chloride is present, and the test should always be repeated before a conclusion is reached. Measurements of sweat sodium concentration are less reliable, but a concentration of greater than 90 mmol/l is in keeping with cystic fibrosis.

There are instances when a false-positive sweat test can occur. The most common of these are listed below.

COMMON CAUSES OF A FALSE POSITIVE SWEAT TEST
Adrenal insufficiency
Anorexia nervosa
Coeliac disease
Hypothyroidism

Case 28

A 55-year-old male smoker with a strong family history of coronary heart disease presents 14 h after a 30 min episode of central crushing chest pain. He was afraid to come to hospital at the time. He is currently pain-free, and his ECG was normal. The A&E officer requests the following test:

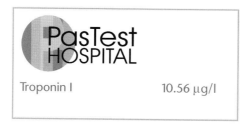

Troponin I   10.56 µg/l

Where should this patient be managed?

Answer 28

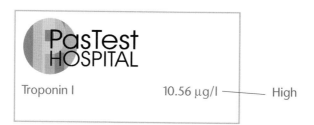

Troponin I   10.56 µg/l ———— High

This patient has a significantly elevated troponin I indicating a significant amount of cardiac damage. The clinical information is consistent with an acute myocardial infarction. The patient is at significant risk of cardiac arrhythmias and should be managed in a coronary care unit.

Case 29

A 77-year-old patient with dementia was admitted generally unwell. No history was obtained. He was pyrexic and appeared a little short of breath. Examination was difficult, although there was the impression of reduced breath sounds at the right lung base. Urinalysis was normal. Blood tests were taken.

PasTest
HOSPITAL

Hb	13.9 g/dl
MCV	95.5 fl
Plt	$188 \times 10^9/l$
WCC	$9.7 \times 10^9/l$
Na$^+$	142 mmol/l
K$^+$	4.4 mmol/l
Urea	4.6 mmol/l
Creatinine	75 μmol/l
Cl$^-$	100 mmol/l
HCO$_3$$^-$	24 mmol/l
CRP	156 mg/l

How do these tests help in the management of this patient?

Answer 29

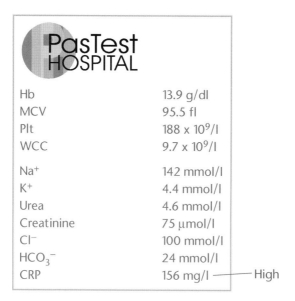

PasTest HOSPITAL	
Hb	13.9 g/dl
MCV	95.5 fl
Plt	188 x 10⁹/l
WCC	9.7 x 10⁹/l
Na⁺	142 mmol/l
K⁺	4.4 mmol/l
Urea	4.6 mmol/l
Creatinine	75 µmol/l
Cl⁻	100 mmol/l
HCO₃⁻	24 mmol/l
CRP	156 mg/l ——— High

Establishing a diagnosis in elderly people can be difficult by clinical assessment alone, especially when no history is available. It is often necessary to place greater emphasis on investigations. Although, in this case, the FBP and U&E are normal, the CRP is significantly raised. In the presence of infection one might expect the WCC to be raised too, but this is not always the case. An infection is likely to be the cause of the patient's illness. A urinary tract infection and pneumonia are the most common causes of these findings in clinical practice. Given the normal urinalysis and examination findings in the chest, pneumonia is the most likely diagnosis.

Case 30

A 38-year-old woman complains of a rash over her face and nose for several weeks and a recent problem with pain and swelling in the joints of her hands. She is married but without children. A number of blood tests were sent – some of which are shown below.

PasTest
HOSPITAL

Hb	11.0 g/dl
MCV	94.4 fl
Plt	128 x 10^9/l
WCC	2.7 x 10^9/l
ESR	77 mm/h
Na^+	136 mmol/l
K^+	4.4 mmol/l
Urea	4.9 mmol/l
Creatinine	64 µmol/l
Cl^-	99 mmol/l
HCO_3^-	26 mmol/l
CRP	7 mg/l
Urinalysis	Protein ++

1. **Summarise the results shown.**

2. **Using the clinical information what is the most likely diagnosis?**

Answer 30

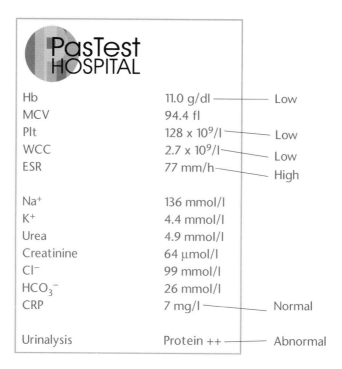

PasTest
HOSPITAL

Hb	11.0 g/dl	Low
MCV	94.4 fl	
Plt	128 x 10⁹/l	Low
WCC	2.7 x 10⁹/l	Low
ESR	77 mm/h	High
Na⁺	136 mmol/l	
K⁺	4.4 mmol/l	
Urea	4.9 mmol/l	
Creatinine	64 µmol/l	
Cl⁻	99 mmol/l	
HCO₃⁻	26 mmol/l	
CRP	7 mg/l	Normal
Urinalysis	Protein ++	Abnormal

1. There are a number of abnormalities on this set of results:

    • the haemoglobin is slightly low

    • the platelet count is slightly below normal

    • the WCC is low

    • the ESR is raised, with a normal CRP

    • protein is noted in the urine.

2. The CRP is normal. This would go against an infectious cause for a raised ESR and be more suggestive of inflammation of some description. There are only a few conditions in which the ESR is elevated but the CRP remains normal. One such condition is systemic lupus erythematosus (SLE) which this patient's clinical features are in keeping with.

Case 31

A 32-year-old diabetic woman is admitted for treatment of a large abscess. The patient is reluctant to undergo surgical intervention and medical treatment is pursued initially. Four days into her care she becomes more unwell and her treatment is changed. A further 3 days on, when her condition remains poor, she agrees to surgical intervention. Below is a chart of her CRP throughout this period.

PasTest
HOSPITAL

DAY	CRP (mg/l)
1	356
2	345
3	387
4	444
5	467
6	499
7	550
8	422
9	302
10	143
11	121

Try to explain the trend in the results.

Answer 31

PasTest
HOSPITAL

DAY	CRP (mg/l)	
1	356	
2	345	
3	387	
4	444	
5	467	
6	499	
7	550	CRP rising until this day; thereafter falling
8	422	
9	302	
10	143	
11	121	

Some of the most rewarding data to interpret are those collated over a period of time when trends can be observed. This scenario illustrates the value of CRP in both supporting a clinical diagnosis and monitoring its response to treatment. On admission this patient's CRP is significantly raised, as one may expect in the presence of an abscess. With the commencement of antibiotics, one might hope for the CRP to improve as the abscess is treated. The worsening of her clinical state and the rising CRP suggest that either the antibiotics are ineffective against the causative organism or they are unable to penetrate the abscess. Day 4 sees a change in treatment, no doubt to an alternative antimicrobial. However, the CRP remains stubbornly high. It is only in the days following surgical intervention that the CRP begins to decrease, reflecting the successful treatment of the abscess.

Case 32

A 58-year-old man complains of an exquisitely tender big toe. It is red, swollen and impossible to examine fully because of pain. No other joints are affected. He has a history of hypertension and a previous myocardial infarction at 49 years of age. He drinks 14 units of alcohol a week. To his knowledge he does not have any kidney problems. Blood tests are shown.

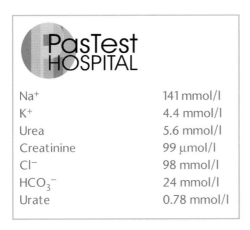

PasTest HOSPITAL

Na^+	141 mmol/l
K^+	4.4 mmol/l
Urea	5.6 mmol/l
Creatinine	99 μmol/l
Cl^-	98 mmol/l
HCO_3^-	24 mmol/l
Urate	0.78 mmol/l

Does this man have gout? Justify your answer.

Answer 32

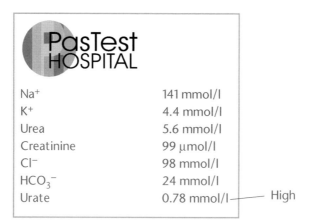

PasTest HOSPITAL	
Na+	141 mmol/l
K+	4.4 mmol/l
Urea	5.6 mmol/l
Creatinine	99 μmol/l
Cl−	98 mmol/l
HCO₃−	24 mmol/l
Urate	0.78 mmol/l —— High

The clinical history is one of podagra (gout of the great toe). The elevated urate in the blood supports this diagnosis. Definitive diagnosis of gout depends on the detection of crystals of sodium urate in synovial fluid (see page 375). However, not all joints with acute gout are amenable to aspiration and one must rely on a clinical impression and supportive blood tests. Remember that the serum urate level can be normal in acute gout.

This patient may well be taking a thiazide diuretic for hypertension. This would place him at higher risk for gout.

Case 33

A 34-year-old woman with acute lymphoblastic leukaemia (ALL) is receiving chemotherapy within the haematology suite of the hospital. Several days into treatment she complains of an intensely sore right knee. On examination there is an effusion and she is unable to extend the knee fully due to pain. She has no pre-existing joint disease. Fluid (35 ml) was aspirated from the knee and sent for analysis along with blood samples.

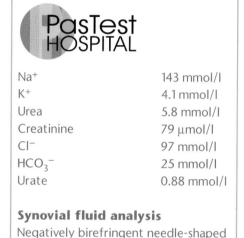

PasTest
HOSPITAL

Na+	143 mmol/l
K+	4.1 mmol/l
Urea	5.8 mmol/l
Creatinine	79 μmol/l
Cl−	97 mmol/l
HCO3−	25 mmol/l
Urate	0.88 mmol/l

Synovial fluid analysis
Negatively birefringent needle-shaped crystals on polarised light microscopy

Interpret these results (see page 375 for details of synovial fluid analysis).

Answer 33

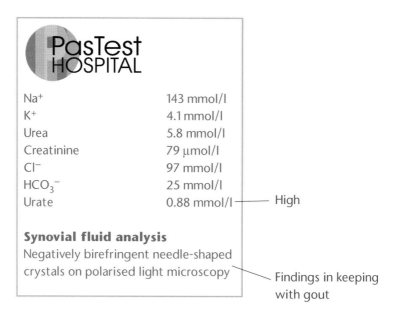

PasTest
HOSPITAL

Na^+	143 mmol/l
K^+	4.1 mmol/l
Urea	5.8 mmol/l
Creatinine	79 µmol/l
Cl^-	97 mmol/l
HCO_3^-	25 mmol/l
Urate	0.88 mmol/l ——— High

Synovial fluid analysis
Negatively birefringent needle-shaped
crystals on polarised light microscopy ——— Findings in keeping
with gout

Hyperuricaemia may occur due to excess purine metabolism. This includes those suffering from haematological malignancies in which there is increased cell turnover, especially following cell lysis from chemotherapy.

The presence of negatively birefringent crystals from the joint aspiration confirms gout.

Case 34

A 67-year-old man attends outpatients with a complaint of constipation and vague abdominal discomfort. Abdominal examination and proctoscopy were normal. Imaging investigations and endoscopy have been arranged. CEA levels were also requested, along with routine blood tests.

PasTest HOSPITAL

Hb	9.1 g/dl
MCV	71.2 fl
Plt	$199 \times 10^9/l$
WCC	$5.6 \times 10^9/l$
Na^+	139 mmol/l
K^+	4.2 mmol/l
Urea	4.5 mmol/l
Creatinine	87 µmol/l
Cl^-	104 mmol/l
HCO_3^-	26 mmol/l
CEA	81 ng/ml

What underlying diagnosis unites all the abnormalities observed?

Answer 34

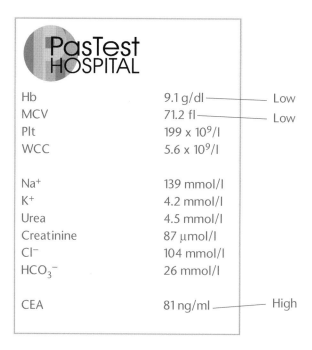

PasTest
HOSPITAL

Hb	9.1 g/dl	Low
MCV	71.2 fl	Low
Plt	199 x 10⁹/l	
WCC	5.6 x 10⁹/l	
Na⁺	139 mmol/l	
K⁺	4.2 mmol/l	
Urea	4.5 mmol/l	
Creatinine	87 µmol/l	
Cl⁻	104 mmol/l	
HCO₃⁻	26 mmol/l	
CEA	81 ng/ml	High

The key findings on this patient's blood tests are a microcytic anaemia (see page 3) and a raised CEA. Given his symptoms, these results should arouse a great deal of suspicion of colorectal carcinoma. Although proctoscopy was normal this visualised only a very small percentage of the large bowel and further imaging is required. In this case the tumour marker merely adds weight to a clinical suspicion.

Case 35

A 55-year-old haemophiliac attends her routine 6-monthly review at hepatology outpatients. She has been attending for several years after contracting hepatitis C from a blood transfusion. The doctor notes that she has not attended for 8 months, and requests a number of blood tests.

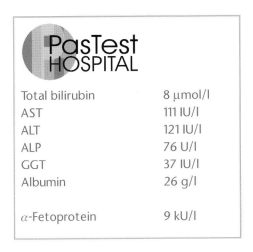

Total bilirubin	8 μmol/l
AST	111 IU/l
ALT	121 IU/l
ALP	76 U/l
GGT	37 IU/l
Albumin	26 g/l
α-Fetoprotein	9 kU/l

What would you infer from these results?

Answer 35

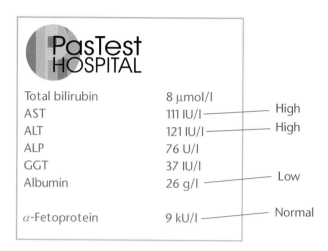

PasTest
HOSPITAL

Total bilirubin	8 µmol/l	
AST	111 IU/l	High
ALT	121 IU/l	High
ALP	76 U/l	
GGT	37 IU/l	
Albumin	26 g/l	Low
α-Fetoprotein	9 kU/l	Normal

This patient most likely has liver cirrhosis secondary to hepatitis C. Her regular attendance at an outpatient clinic is at least in part for surveillance for hepatocellular carcinoma. Her α-fetoprotein level is within normal limits, indicating a low likelihood of this tumour being present. Generally ultrasound of the liver will be used in conjunction with α-fetoprotein measurements to seek out a hepatocellular carcinoma. A significant percentage of tumour markers are performed for monitoring so you should expect to interpret some normal results.

Case 36

A 44-year-old reformed IV drug user with known hepatitis C is well known to the local hepatologists. He has been attending on a regular basis and is enrolled in the hepatocellular carcinoma surveillance programme. Below are an overview of his blood tests.

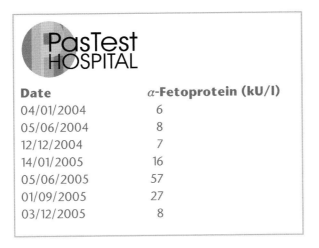

Date	α-Fetoprotein (kU/l)
04/01/2004	6
05/06/2004	8
12/12/2004	7
14/01/2005	16
05/06/2005	57
01/09/2005	27
03/12/2005	8

What may explain the pattern in these results?

Answer 36

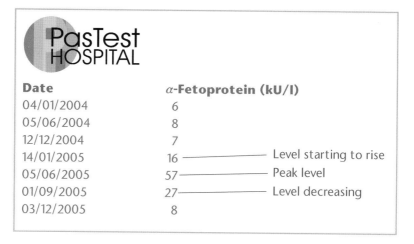

PasTest HOSPITAL

Date	α-Fetoprotein (kU/l)	
04/01/2004	6	
05/06/2004	8	
12/12/2004	7	
14/01/2005	16	Level starting to rise
05/06/2005	57	Peak level
01/09/2005	27	Level decreasing
03/12/2005	8	

One important role of α-fetoprotein measurement is demonstrated well in this patient with hepatitis C. It is one of the more specific tumour markers and can be used with some degree of confidence to monitor patients with liver cirrhosis who have a substantially increased risk of developing hepatocellular carcinoma (HCC). Identifying a patient who has developed HCC early may allow successful treatment to be instigated, as opposed to when it is identified because of symptoms. The level in January 2005 is higher than 6 months previously but is not dramatically elevated. However, 6 months later it has increased substantially. This suggests the development of HCC, and ultrasound and/or other cross-sectional imaging would be merited. The encouraging downward trend in the following 6 months would indicate that the tumour has been successfully treated.

Case 37

A 55-year-old senior civil servant plucks up the courage to attend his GP after complaints of a poor urinary stream, frequency and nocturia. He is concerned as his father had 'prostate problems', On rectal examination an enlarged prostate was felt. Later that week his renal function and prostate-specific antigen tests come back.

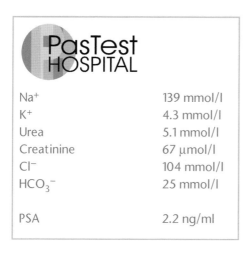

PasTest
HOSPITAL

Na^+	139 mmol/l
K^+	4.3 mmol/l
Urea	5.1 mmol/l
Creatinine	67 µmol/l
Cl^-	104 mmol/l
HCO_3^-	25 mmol/l
PSA	2.2 ng/ml

Does this patient have anything to worry about?

Answer 37

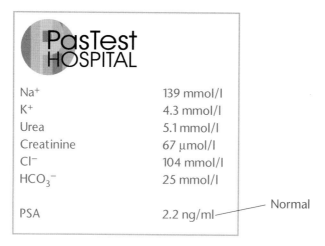

PasTest
HOSPITAL

Na$^+$	139 mmol/l
K$^+$	4.3 mmol/l
Urea	5.1 mmol/l
Creatinine	67 µmol/l
Cl$^-$	104 mmol/l
HCO$_3^-$	25 mmol/l
PSA	2.2 ng/ml — Normal

Of all the tumour markers available, probably the most commonly requested is PSA. It is sometimes used in an attempt to identify the presence of prostatic carcinoma, but more usefully in monitoring the disease and treatment response. This patient has obstructive urinary symptoms and an enlarged prostate, but this does not mean that he has prostate carcinoma. Likewise a normal PSA does not exclude the presence of this tumour. However, this man most likely has benign prostatic hypertrophy. There are a number of causes of a raised PSA, as shown below.

CAUSES OF RAISED PSA

Prostate carcinoma
Instrumentation of prostate (including urinary catheterisation)
Urinary tract infection
Recent ejaculation

Case 38

A 28-year-old media studies student attends A&E with a swollen left testicle. He is sexually active, with multiple sexual partners in the last 6 months. The A&E officer is concerned, and arranges admission. Ultrasound of the scrotum and blood tests were requested.

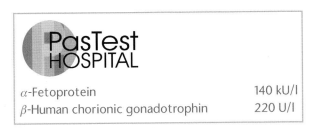

α-Fetoprotein	140 kU/l
β-Human chorionic gonadotrophin	220 U/l

Can these results be explained by a diagnosis of epididymo-orchitis?

Answer 38

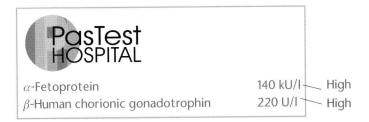

α-Fetoprotein	140 kU/l	High
β-Human chorionic gonadotrophin	220 U/l	High

α-Fetoprotein is one of the few tumour markers with a good specificity for two different tumours – hepatocellular carcinoma and testicular teratoma. Similarly testicular teratoma is unique in characteristically causing high levels of two tumour markers – α-fetoprotein and β-hCG. Both tumour markers are significantly elevated here indicating a high probability of testicular malignancy. Following treatment, these markers should be checked again and should have decreased.

Case 39

A 55-year-old woman is admitted under the surgeons with a distended abdomen. She admits that it has become increasingly large over the past few weeks, but was scared to come to hospital. She has no complaints of abdominal pain and her bowel habit is normal. The enthusiastic junior doctor who admitted the patient included in the notes she has sent blood for CEA, CA-125 and CA-19-9.

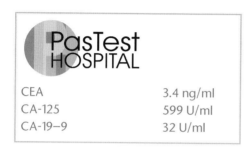

CEA	3.4 ng/ml
CA-125	599 U/ml
CA-19–9	32 U/ml

What do these blood results tell you?

Answer 39

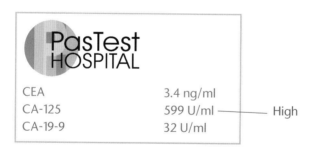

CEA	3.4 ng/ml
CA-125	599 U/ml —— High
CA-19-9	32 U/ml

It is not uncommon (though not particularly good practice), especially in puzzling clinical cases, to request a host of blood tests. Tumour markers for intra-abdominal pathology are sometimes used in this manner. However, due to the non-specific nature of these results, abnormal results can sometimes add to the diagnostic conundrum. The abnormal marker in this case is CA-125. This is most closely associated with ovarian malignancy. The clinical history is certainly in keeping with this, as the distended abdomen may reflect both tumour bulk and/or the presence of malignant ascites.

ENDOCRINOLOGY

3

ENDOCRINOLOGY

Endocrine disorders can be divided into primary and secondary disorders. In a primary endocrine gland disorder, the problem lies within the endocrine gland itself. Thus in primary hyperthyroidism, the principal problem is an overactive thyroid gland. Secondary endocrine diseases arise when there is a problem with the hormones controlling the activity of the target gland, such as the overproduction of a hormone by the pituitary gland.

Thyroid hormones

Normally, thyrotrophin-releasing hormone (TRH) is released from the hypothalamus and stimulates the pituitary gland to release thyroid-stimulating hormone (TSH). This hormone then acts on the thyroid gland and results in the liberation of thyroxine (T_4) and triiodothyronine (T_3) into the circulation. These hormones exert negative feedback on both the hypothalamus and pituitary, and result in a reduction in the production of TRH and TSH. Most of the T_3 and T_4 in the body is carried by carrier proteins (principally thyroxine-binding globulin, TBG). A small percentage is present in unbound form, and it is this that is physiologically active. In clinical practice, the commonly measured hormones are TSH, free T_4, and T_3. Total T_4 (ie bound and unbound forms) is sometimes given.

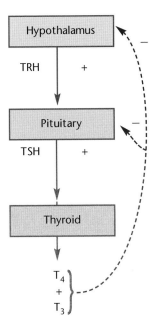

Fig 3.1

Hyperthyroidism

In primary hyperthyroidism (eg with Graves' disease), the thyroid gland autonomously produces thyroid hormones. The levels of T_3 and T_4 therefore rise. Normal negative feedback continues, and the level of TSH will be low. In T_3 thyrotoxicosis, the T_3 level may be elevated in isolation.

In secondary hyperthyroidism (eg due to a pituitary tumour secreting TSH), the levels of T_3 and T_4 will again be high, but this time the TSH level will be inappropriately normal or high.

> The finding of a normal TSH level in the setting of raised T_3 and T_4 should raise suspicions of a pituitary lesion, since in normal circumstances the TSH level will be suppressed

Hypothyroidism

In primary hypothyroidism (eg with Hashimoto's thyroiditis), the thyroid gland is defective. The levels of T_3 and T_4 are low. As a result of reduced negative feedback, the TSH level will be high.

In secondary hypothyroidism (eg destructive pituitary tumour), the levels of T_3 and T_4 will again be low, but this is because of low TSH levels.

Sick euthyroid syndrome

Caution should be taken when interpreting thyroid function tests in a patient with an acute illness. This is because thyroid function tests are often abnormal during the acute phase of an illness, but normalise on its resolution. This phenomenon is known as the sick euthyroid syndrome, indicating that the patient is euthyroid (ie normal thyroid function), but that he or she has an intercurrent illness. The common picture in sick euthyroid syndrome is one of low T_3 and T_4 with low or normal TSH.

> Be cautious when interpreting thyroid function tests in an acutely unwell patient.

SUMMARY OF HORMONE CHANGES IN VARIOUS THYROID DISEASE STATES		
	T_3/T_4	TSH
Primary hyperthyroidism	↑	↓
T_3 thyrotoxicosis	Only T_3 ↑	↓
Secondary hyperthyroidism	↑	↑
Primary hypothyroidism	↓	↑
Secondary hypothyroidism	↓	↓
Sick euthyroid syndrome	↓	↓

Variations in Thyroxine Binding Globulin (TBG) levels

Care must be taken when interpreting free and total T_4 levels. This is because the level of TBG can vary in various states. Always remember that it is the level of free hormone that is important physiologically. Factors influencing the level of TBG are listed below.

INCREASE TBG	DECREASE TBG
High oestrogen states, eg pregnancy, oral contraceptive pill use	High corticosteroid levels
Hypothyroidism	Protein deficiency states: low intake (malnutrition); low synthesis (chronic liver disease); increased losses (nephrotic syndrome)
	Thyrotoxicosis

Adrenal hormones

Normally, corticotrophin-releasing hormone (CRH) is released from the hypothalamus and stimulates the pituitary gland to release adrenocorticotrophic hormone (ACTH). This hormone then acts on the adrenal cortex and results in the release of glucocorticoids. Glucocorticoids exert negative feedback on both the hypothalamus and pituitary, and result in a reduction in the production of CRH and ACTH.

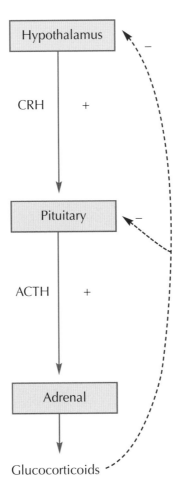

Fig 3.2

Cushing's syndrome

Cushing's syndrome results from glucocorticoid excess. It is seen most commonly in patients receiving glucocorticoid treatment, eg for chronic severe asthma. Endogenous forms of Cushing's syndrome have several causes which are listed below.

ENDOGENOUS CAUSES OF CUSHING'S SYNDROME

Primary adrenal disease
- Adrenal tumour (adenoma or carcinoma)

ACTH excess
- From the pituitary gland (Cushing's disease)
- From an ACTH-producing tumour

In primary adrenal disease causing Cushing's syndrome, the adrenal gland autonomously produces adrenal hormones. Normal negative feedback continues, and the level of ACTH will be low.

In instances of secondary hyperadrenalism (eg due to a pituitary tumour), the ACTH level will be normal or high.

There are two main methods for diagnosing Cushing's syndrome:

1. The 24-h urinary free cortisol level

An elevated level of steroid in the urine is in keeping with Cushing's syndrome.

2. Dexamethasone suppression tests

Normally, if a person is given a dose of dexamethasone, it has a negative feedback effect on the adrenal axis, resulting in low circulating levels of cortisol. Two variants of this test are used:

i. Overnight dexamethasone suppression test

The patient is given 1 mg of dexamethasone at 11.00 pm, and blood is taken at 9.00 am the following morning. Cortisol levels of more than 100 nmol/l are abnormal, and should raise suspicion of Cushing's syndrome.

ii. Low-dose dexamethasone suppression test

The patient is given repeated doses of dexamethasone (8 x 0.5 mg doses at 6 h intervals) starting at 9.00 am. Cortisol levels of more than 50 nmol/l 48 h after the first dose are abnormal, and suggestive of Cushing's syndrome.

Other specialised tests can be carried out in an attempt to differentiate between the causes of Cushing's syndrome.

Hypoadrenalism

In primary hypoadrenalism (eg Addison's disease), the adrenal gland itself is defective. As a result of reduced negative feedback, the ACTH level will be high.

In secondary hypoadrenalism, ACTH levels will be low.

Short Synacthen® test

Synacthen®, or SYNthetic ACTH, is used to stimulate the adrenal gland. Normally, an injection of Synacthen® will result in an increase in circulating cortisol levels. If the patient has a primary adrenal disease, the Synacthen® will not have its normal effect, and the rise in cortisol levels will be poor. A cortisol level of less than 600 nmol/l 30 min after Synacthen® has been administered is in keeping with failure of the adrenal gland. The Synacthen® test will be normal in cases of secondary hypoadrenalism.

Insulin tolerance test

This test is used in specialist centres to assess adrenal function as well as to assess for growth hormone deficiency.

Several criteria must be met before this test can be attempted.

CRITERIA TO BE MET BEFORE PERFORMING AN INSULIN TOLERANCE TEST

Cortisol level > 100 nmol/l
Normal thyroid function
No cardiovascular disease
No epilepsy or other seizure activity or blackouts

The essence of the test is to induce hypoglycaemia (blood glucose must fall to less than 2.2 mmol/l) in a carefully controlled environment. In a normal patient, a stress response will occur with a rise in cortisol and growth hormone levels. Normally, the cortisol level should rise to more than 550 nmol/l, and the growth hormone level to more than 20 mU/l.

Phaeochromocytoma

These tumours are associated with excess circulating catecholamines. Diagnosis relies on the demonstration of excessive amounts of catecholamine breakdown products (metanephrines) in the urine. Generally three negative tests are required before the diagnosis can be excluded.

The thirst axis

Psychogenic polydipsia and diabetes insipidus

The combination of passing excessive volumes of urine (polyuria) with excessive thirst (polydipsia) is common. The water deprivation test is used to differentiate between two major causes – psychogenic polydipsia and diabetes insipidus (DI).

Patients with psychogenic polydipsia simply drink fluid in excess for psychological or psychiatric reasons.

In DI, there is a problem with antidiuretic hormone (ADH). ADH normally acts on the collecting ducts in the kidney to stimulate water reabsorption. If ADH does not function properly, too much urine is passed. In turn the patient becomes relatively dehydrated and drinks to compensate for this.

MEMORY AID

Diuretic medications increase urine volume

Therefore, antidiuretic hormone (ADH) does the opposite, and acts to conserve water

There are two forms of DI – cranial and nephrogenic. In cranial DI, there is a problem with the release of ADH from the hypothalamus. Blood levels of ADH are low. In nephrogenic DI, there is sufficient ADH in the system, but it fails to exert its effects on the kidney.

The water deprivation test restricts patients' intake of water. If they have psychogenic polydipsia, reducing water intake will solve their problem and they will gradually return to normal. However, with DI, water restriction will result in a worsening state of dehydration.

The test involves forbidding the patient to drink after waking. Blood and urine osmolalities are tested each hour for a period of 8 h. In health (or psychogenic polydipsia), one would expect the patient to retain water and to pass concentrated urine (with a high urine osmolality). In DI, the urine osmolality does not rise, and the patient becomes dehydrated with a rise in serum osmolality.

To differentiate between the two forms of DI, patients are then given a dose of a synthetic ADH compound called desmopressin. This will correct the problem in cranial DI, but will have no effect in nephrogenic DI.

Syndrome of inappropriate ADH secretion (SIADH)

In this condition, there is a state of excessive ADH production. SIADH has many causes, the most common of which are listed in the table.

COMMON CAUSES OF SIADH	

Intrathoracic causes:
   • Infection
   • Tumour
Intracranial causes:
   • Infection
   • Tumour
   • Head injury
	Medications:
	   • Carbamazepine
	   • Antipsychotics

SIADH is, in essence, the opposite of DI. Excessive ADH action results in retention of water, with the subsequent development of dilute serum and concentrated urine.

For a person to be labelled with the diagnosis of SIADH the following criteria should be met:

1. Normal renal function

2. Normal adrenal function (assess using a short Synacthen® test)

3. Normal thyroid function

4. Hyponatraemia

5. Low serum osmolality

6. Urine osmolality greater than serum osmolality

7. Urinary sodium excretion more than 50 mmol/l

8. Absence of dehydration or fluid overload.

Hyperprolactinaemia

There are many causes of a raised serum prolactin level (see box below). Very high levels (>5000 mU/l) strongly suggest a prolactin-secreting pituitary tumour.

COMMON CAUSES OF HYPERPROLACTINAEMIA

Physiological:
- Pregnancy
- Lactation

Prolactin-secreting pituitary tumour

Medications:
- Phenothiazine antipsychotics
- Most antiemetics

Polycystic ovarian syndrome

Following a seizure

Primary hypothyroidism

Hyperglycaemia

The diagnosis of diabetes mellitus and related hyperglycaemic states relies on accurate interpretation of blood glucose readings. A patient's glycaemic status can be classed as one of the following:

- Normal

- Impaired fasting glucose

- Impaired glucose tolerance

- Diabetes mellitus

- Gestational diabetes mellitus.

In some circumstances, diabetes will be suspected clinically, particularly if the patient is symptomatic from hyperglycaemia. In other instances, hyperglycaemia will be detected incidentally when a blood glucose level is checked. Typical symptoms are shown in the box below.

SYMPTOMS OF DIABETES MELLITUS

Polyuria
Polydipsia
Weight loss
Fatigue
Blurring of vision
Symptoms related to a complication of diabetes such as a cutaneous abscess

An oral glucose tolerance test (OGTT) is often used in differentiating between these various states. This test involves giving the patient a 75 g glucose load by mouth, after they have been fasting. Plasma glucose level is measured at baseline and after 2 h.

Diabetes mellitus may be diagnosed in a variety of ways. Any one of the following is sufficient:

1. A single random plasma glucose of more than 11.1 mmol/l in a patient with symptoms

2. Two separate random plasma glucose samples of more than 11.1 mmol/l in a patient without symptoms

3. A single fasting plasma glucose of more than 7.0 mmol/l in a patient with symptoms

4. Two separate fasting plasma glucose samples of more than 7.0 mmol/l in a patient without symptoms

5. A plasma glucose level of 11.1 mmol/l or more 2 h after a glucose load in an OGTT. An OGTT is generally only performed if borderline results are obtained on random or fasting samples.

> If a patient is asymptomatic, two blood tests are required before diabetes mellitus can be diagnosed

Patients with **normoglycaemia** (ie definitely not diabetic) have a fasting plasma glucose of less than 6.1 mmol/l. Two hours following a glucose load in an OGTT, the plasma glucose will be less than 7.8 mmol/l.

'Impaired fasting glucose' and **'impaired glucose tolerance'** are terms used to describe states of glycaemic control that lie somewhere between normal and frank diabetes mellitus. The terms are not mutually exclusive. It is therefore possible for a patient to have both impaired fasting glucose and impaired glucose tolerance. Alternatively, they may have one or other of the terms attached to them in isolation. The significance of labelling a patient with one of these terms lies with the fact that such patients have an increased risk of developing diabetes mellitus in the future. The diagnostic criteria are shown in the table below.

	NORMAL	IMPAIRED FASTING	IMPAIRED GLUCOSE TOLERANCE	DIABETES MELLITUS
Fasting plasma glucose (mmol/l)	<6.1	6.1–6.9	Not necessary for diagnosis	≥7.0
Plasma glucose 2 hours after glucose load in OGTT (mmol/l)	<7.8	Not necessary for diagnosis	7.8–11.0	≥11.1

Gestational diabetes mellitus describes diabetes that is of new onset in pregnancy, or that is first noted during pregnancy. The principles of diagnosis are identical to those above. The term may be used if a woman fits the criteria for impaired glucose tolerance or diabetes mellitus while pregnant. All such women should have an OGTT at least 6 weeks following delivery, and be re-classified as necessary. The significance of gestational diabetes mellitus again relates to the fact that such patients have an increased chance of developing diabetes mellitus in later life.

Glycated haemoglobin

Random blood glucose measurements are useful for monitoring variations on a day-to-day basis, however, the inevitable variation makes interpretation of long-term trends difficult. For this reason measurement of glycated haemoglobin (HbA1 or HbA1$_C$) is often used.

Glycated haemoglobin is the product of the reaction between glucose and haemoglobin A (the main type of haemoglobin in most adults). The higher the average blood glucose level, the higher the glycated haemoglobin level will be. Since red blood cells have an average life-span of around 60 days, glycated haemoglobin estimation provides information on the glycaemic control over this time period.

The Diabetes Control and Complications Trial (DCCT) provided evidence that well-controlled diabetes was associated with fewer microvascular complications (*N Engl J Med* 1993; **329**(14): 977–986). For most patients, a target HbA1$_C$ of between 6.5 and 7.5% will be adequate. A slightly less ambitious target of between 7 and 8% may prove adequate for some patients, and reduce the risk of hypoglycaemic attacks when compared with a more intensive treatment regimen.

Glycated haemoglobin is reliable only when normal haemoglobin is present in red blood cells that have normal life-spans. If a haemoglobin disorder is present, or in patients who have red cells with shortened life-spans (eg haemolytic anaemia), measurement of fructosamine levels may be used instead to measure glycaemic control. Fructosamine is a glycated plasma protein, and provides information on glucose levels over the previous 1–3 weeks.

Hypoglycaemia

Hypoglycaemia describes a plasma glucose that is lower than normal (less than 3.5 mmol/l). The commonest cause is an imbalance between intake and insulin requirements in a patient with type 1 diabetes mellitus (eg the patient who takes normal insulin without eating lunch). Other causes of hypoglycaemia are listed in the box below.

CAUSES OF HYPOGLYCAEMIA

Imbalance between insulin and calorie intake in type 1 diabetes
Excess exogenous insulin administration
As a side-effect of anti-hyperglycaemic medication
Insulinoma
Liver failure
Alcohol ingestion

A fairly common clinical scenario is the patient who presents with hypoglycaemia of unknown cause. Endogenous insulin (ie insulin derived from an insulinoma) can be differentiated easily from exogenous insulin (ie a patient with Munchausen's syndrome who administers insulin to themselves in an attempt to seek medical attention) with a little knowledge of insulin physiology.

Normal physiological insulin is manufactured in the body from proinsulin which in turn is derived from pre-proinsulin. Each protein precursor is cleaved to yield its product. This cleavage process generates a 'waste' chain of amino acids called C-peptide.

If hypoglycaemia is due to excess endogenous insulin from an insulinoma, one would expect high insulin and C-peptide levels in a patient who is hypoglycaemic.

Exogenous insulin does not contain C-peptide. Therefore, a hypoglycaemic patient with raised levels of insulin in the blood but normal/low levels of C-peptide is likely to have been administered insulin.

Acromegaly

Acromegaly is associated with an elevated level of growth hormone (GH), usually due to a pituitary tumour. Measuring the level is not a reliable method of making this diagnosis. Insulin-like growth factor-I (IGF-I) levels can be used as a marker of average GH levels and, if raised, are suggestive of acromegaly. The definitive test for the diagnosis is a glucose tolerance test, exactly like that used in the investigation of hyperglycaemia. The test is performed in the same manner, but GH levels are measured. Failure of the GH level to fall below 1m U/l is in keeping with a diagnosis of acromegaly.

Acromegaly is diagnosed if the GH level is >1 m U/l during a glucose tolerance test

Case 40

A 64-year-old woman is admitted with palpitations. She feels that these have been intermittent over the last month. Examination reveals an anxious woman with an irregularly irregular pulse at 120 beats per minute. ECG confirms the suspicions of atrial fibrillation. As part of her initial investigations, the following blood test is returned.

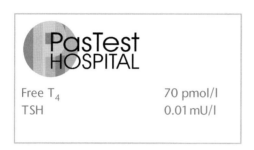

PasTest
HOSPITAL

Free T_4 70 pmol/l
TSH   0.01 mU/l

What is the underlying cause of the atrial fibrillation?

Answer 40

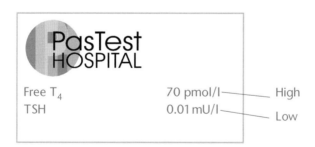

PasTest
HOSPITAL

Free T_4 70 pmol/l —————— High
TSH   0.01 mU/l —————— Low

This woman has primary hyperthyroidism. Her overactive thyroid gland is producing thyroid hormones in excess. Normal negative feedback mechanisms still function, however, so the TSH level is suppressed.

It is not uncommon for atrial fibrillation to be the only evidence of hyperthyroidism, so always remember to check thyroid function in such patients.

Case 41

A patient is reviewed at the chest clinic. He was treated over one year ago for pulmonary tuberculosis. He now complains of lethargy. Clinical examination reveals no chest abnormalities, but he is found to have significant postural hypotension. A urea and electrolyte (U&E) blood test is sent and, on the basis of the results, the following test is arranged.

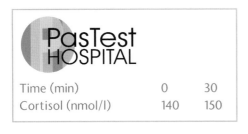

Time (min)	0	30
Cortisol (nmol/l)	140	150

1. **What is the test, and what does it demonstrate in this case?**

2. **What were the likely abnormalities on the U&E that raised suspicions of this disorder?**

3. **What is the likely underlying disease?**

Answer 41

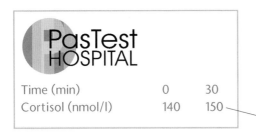

Time (min)	0	30
Cortisol (nmol/l)	140	150

Poor rise in cortisol post-injection with Synacthen®

1. This is a short Synacthen® test. The cortisol level fails to rise to more than 600 nmol/l 30 min after injection with Synacthen®. This indicates primary hypoadrenalism (ie a problem with the adrenal gland itself).

2. A low sodium and raised potassium level are commonly found. The glucose level would also be expected to be low.

3. The underlying disease is primary hypoadrenalism, likely due to autoimmune adrenalitis or tuberculosis affecting the adrenal gland.

Case 42

A patient is referred to the endocrine clinic complaining of excess thirst and of passing excessive amounts of urine. A random blood glucose level is 4.2 mmol/l. He is admitted to hospital and a water deprivation test is arranged. The results are shown.

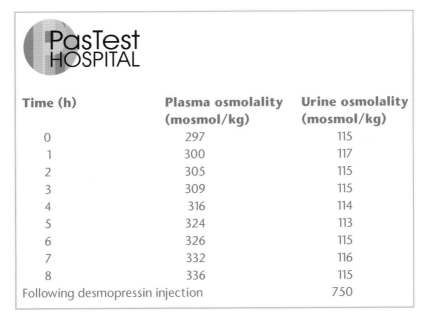

PasTest HOSPITAL

Time (h)	Plasma osmolality (mosmol/kg)	Urine osmolality (mosmol/kg)
0	297	115
1	300	117
2	305	115
3	309	115
4	316	114
5	324	113
6	326	115
7	332	116
8	336	115
Following desmopressin injection		750

1. **What is your interpretation of the blood glucose level?**

2. **What is the diagnosis?**

Answer 42

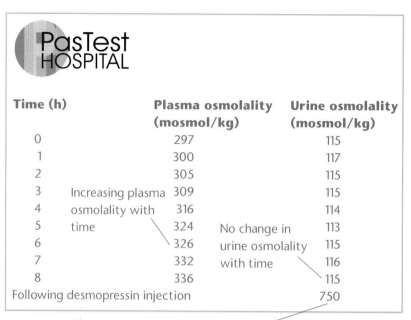

Time (h)		Plasma osmolality (mosmol/kg)		Urine osmolality (mosmol/kg)
0		297		115
1		300		117
2		305		115
3	Increasing plasma	309		115
4	osmolality with	316		114
5	time	324	No change in	113
6		326	urine osmolality	115
7		332	with time	116
8		336		115
Following desmopressin injection				750

Increase in urine osmolality following
desmopressin injection

1. The random blood glucose level is normal. The patient therefore does not have diabetes mellitus. It is important to exclude this diagnosis, since it can also present with polydipsia and polyuria.

2. The diagnosis is cranial diabetes insipidus. The patient has a problem producing ADH. When deprived of water, he is unable to concentrate the urine. The plasma rapidly becomes more concentrated. Following an injection of synthetic ADH (desmopressin), the urine osmolality increases. This shows that the kidney is still sensitive to the effects of ADH, and excludes nephrogenic diabetes insipidus as the diagnosis.

Case 43

A patient is referred to the endocrine clinic after having been assessed in eye A&E. The registrar arranges for a glucose tolerance test to be carried out.

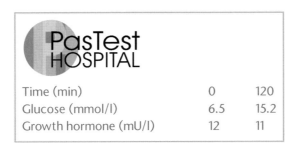

Time (min)	0	120
Glucose (mmol/l)	6.5	15.2
Growth hormone (mU/l)	12	11

1. **What two diagnoses can be made on the basis of this test?**

2. **Why do you think the patient was seen in eye A&E?**

Answer 43

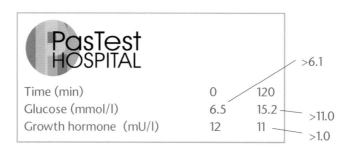

PasTest
HOSPITAL

			>6.1
Time (min)	0	120	
Glucose (mmol/l)	6.5	15.2	>11.0
Growth hormone (mU/l)	12	11	>1.0

1. The two diagnoses that can be made from this one test are: diabetes
    mellitus and acromegaly.

    The glucose level before the start of the test is elevated in keeping with the
    label of impaired fasting glucose. However, the abnormally high glucose level
    2 h after the glucose load confirms the diagnosis of diabetes mellitus.

    The growth hormone level is greater than 2.0 µg/l at all stages of the test,
    allowing the diagnosis of acromegaly to be made.

2. The commonest cause of acromegaly is a pituitary tumour. This commonly
    extends in an upwards direction and can compress the optic chiasma causing
    a bitemporal hemianopia. Loss of temporal visual fields is the probable
    reason for presentation at eye A&E.

Case 44

A 21-year-old woman is referred to the medical clinic because of abnormal thyroid function results noted by her GP. There is no personal or family history of thyroid disease, and she is on no medication, but the GP requested the test because the patient had been feeling generally unwell recently. Clinical examination is unremarkable. The thyroid function tests are repeated and the following results are obtained.

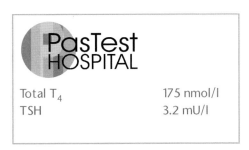

PasTest HOSPITAL

Total T_4	175 nmol/l
TSH	3.2 mU/l

1. **How would you interpret these tests?**

2. **What two tests should be ordered?**

Answer 44

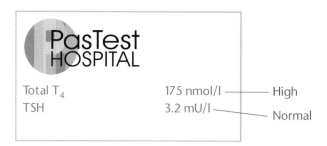

PasTest
HOSPITAL

Total T_4	175 nmol/l	High
TSH	3.2 mU/l	Normal

1. Care should be taken when interpreting these results. Note that the TOTAL T_4 level is given, not the FREE T_4 level. It is the free level that is important physiologically. It is impossible to make any further comments on these tests other than to say that the total T_4 level is raised, and the TSH is normal.

2. First, the free T_4 level should be measured. In this case it was normal (result not shown), indicating normal thyroid function. The patient therefore has an elevated total T_4 level with a normal free T_4 level. The reason for this is increased levels of TBG. The most likely reason for this is a high oestrogen state (eg pregnancy or use of the oral contraceptive pill). Since the question states that the patient is not on any medication, the most likely diagnosis here is pregnancy. The second test that should be performed is therefore a pregnancy test.

Case 45

A 57-year-old man is referred to the hypertension clinic. Two tests are performed in order to screen for an endocrine cause of hypertension.

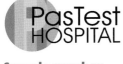

PasTest
HOSPITAL

Sample number	Urine metanephrines (μmol/day)
1	2.1
2	2.6
3	2.1

Blood cortisol	225 nmol/l at 9.00 am following 1 mg dexamethasone at 11.00 pm the evening before

How would you interpret these results?

Answer 45

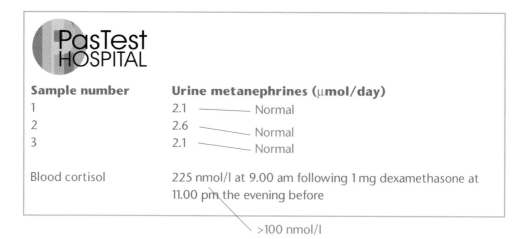

PasTest HOSPITAL

Sample number	Urine metanephrines (μmol/day)
1	2.1 ————— Normal
2	2.6 ————— Normal
3	2.1 ————— Normal

Blood cortisol — 225 nmol/l at 9.00 am following 1 mg dexamethasone at 11.00 pm the evening before

>100 nmol/l

Three separate 24-h urine collections for urinary metanephrines have been taken. The metanephrine levels are normal in each. This excludes phaeochromocytoma as a cause of the hypertension with some certainty.

The second test shows the results of an overnight dexamethasone suppression test. The morning cortisol level is greater than 100 nmol/l, suggesting a diagnosis of Cushing's syndrome.

TOXICOLOGY

4

TOXICOLOGY

Poisoning is one of the commonest causes of admission to hospital. It is most commonly deliberate, but can also be accidental, sometimes due to the accumulation of prescribed medications.

The management of a poisoned patient largely involves supportive care, allowing the body to excrete or metabolise the drug naturally. In certain circumstances, antidotes may be necessary along with other modalities designed to clear the drug more quickly from the body.

Data interpretation in a poisoned patient relies mainly on the correct interpretation of blood levels and urine screening tests.

Paracetamol overdose

One of the commonest drugs taken in overdose is paracetamol. This reflects its ready availability and ubiquitous use.

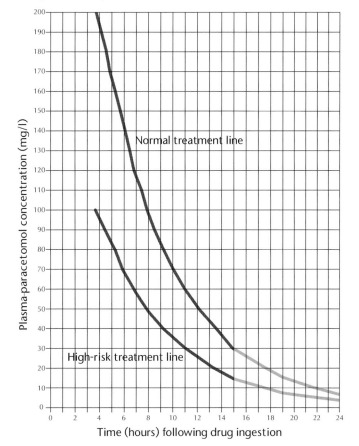

Fig 4.1:

When taken in overdose, paracetamol depletes antioxidant stores in hepatocytes, and can result in liver damage. Administration of the antidote *N*-acetylcysteine (NAC) can augment these stores and reduce or prevent liver damage. However, NAC administration is not without its problems, for example there is a risk of anaphylaxis. It is therefore not routinely given to all patients who have taken paracetamol in excess. In order to decide who should receive NAC, the normogram Fig 4.1 should be used. This can be found in the *British National Formulary* (BNF).

It is critical to know when the paracetamol was taken, and to measure the blood level at least 4 h after this time. In suspected major overdoses (greater than 12 g), NAC may be given presumptively on presentation, but blood levels should always be checked after 4 h.

DON'T FORGET

Always check plasma paracetamol levels at least 4 h after ingestion

---

One will note the two lines on the graph. In routine circumstances, use the normal treatment line. Plot the blood concentration of paracetamol against the time following ingestion and compare this point to the treatment line. If it is on or above the line, treatment should be given. If it is below, there is no indication for treatment. Some patients are deemed 'high risk' for liver damage, and for them the 'high-risk treatment line' should be used. Such patients are presumed to have lower than normal antioxidant stores.

PATIENTS AT HIGH RISK IN PARACETAMOL OVERDOSE

On prescribed hepatic enzyme-inducing drugs
(eg phenytoin, rifampicin, carbamazepine)
Alcoholics
Malnutrition (including anorexia nervosa)
Patients with AIDS

MEMORY AID

Always assess paracetamol overdose patients for high-risk status

---

Drugs with a low therapeutic ratio

The therapeutic ratio is the ratio between the dose of a drug needed to cause a toxic effect and the dose required to produce the intended effect. Drugs with a low therapeutic ratio thus have a small difference between helpful blood levels for treatment and toxic levels. The plasma levels of such medications can be easily measured.

EXAMPLES OF DRUGS WITH NARROW THERAPEUTIC RATIOS

Digoxin
Theophylline
Lithium
Phenytoin
Antibiotics, eg gentamicin, vancomycin, tobramycin

Urine testing for drug metabolites

A number of drugs can be detected in urine. A urine drug screen is often requested when a patient presents with unusual symptoms and there is a suspicion of potential drug use.

TYPICAL COMPONENTS OF URINE 'DRUGS' SCREEN

Amphetamines, barbiturates, benzodiazepines, methadone, cannabinoids, cocaine metabolites, LSD and opiates

Case 46

A 72 year-old woman is admitted complaining of poor appetite, nausea and vomiting. She also complains of intermittent palpitations and visual disturbance. She had a stomach upset one week previously and had been off her food and consumed little fluid. Her medical history includes hypertension, atrial fibrillation and vertigo. She is unable to recall her medications. An ECG was reported as having ST-segment abnormalities, but the house officer did not feel that this was significant.

PasTest HOSPITAL

Hb	12.5 g/dl
MCV	95.7 fl
Plt	293 x 10^9/l
WCC	6.7 x 10^9/l
Na$^+$	139 mmol/l
K$^+$	3.1 mmol/l
Urea	15.6 mmol/l
Creatinine	298 μmol/l
Cl$^-$	104 mmol/l
HCO$_3^-$	27 mmol/l
Digoxin level	2.9 nmol/l

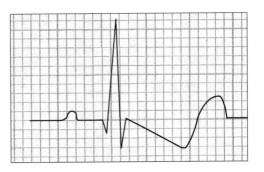

Explain the full significance of these results.

Answer 46

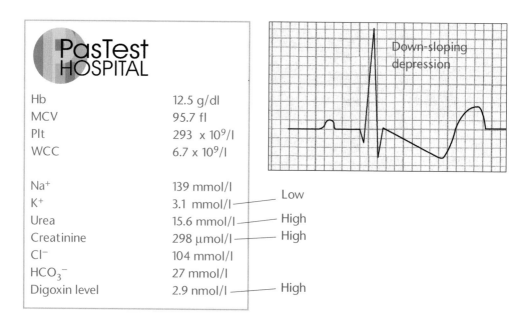

PasTest HOSPITAL

Hb	12.5 g/dl	
MCV	95.7 fl	
Plt	293 x 10⁹/l	
WCC	6.7 x 10⁹/l	
Na⁺	139 mmol/l	
K⁺	3.1 mmol/l	Low
Urea	15.6 mmol/l	High
Creatinine	298 μmol/l	High
Cl⁻	104 mmol/l	
HCO₃⁻	27 mmol/l	
Digoxin level	2.9 nmol/l	High

ECG label: Down-sloping depression

This patient has been prescribed digoxin for atrial fibrillation, and has digoxin toxicity. Digoxin is a drug with a narrow therapeutic ratio and a normal therapeutic range of 0.8–2.0 nmol/l. A level as high as 2.9 nmol/l is enough for the symptoms described in this elderly patient. Digoxin levels can accumulate rapidly in patients with renal impairment. It is likely that this woman has become dehydrated following a bout of gastroenteritis. Renal impairment has caused the rise in plasma digoxin resulting in toxicity. Hypokalaemia is also present. This can exacerbate the symptoms of digoxin toxicity.

This iatrogenic problem is simply treated. Fluid resuscitation with the replacement of potassium intravenously and the exclusion of digoxin is appropriate in this case. The ECG shows down-sloping ST-segment depression ('reverse tick') often seen in patients on digoxin, and would have been a clue here that the patient was taking this drug.

Case 47

A 20-year-old law student attends A&E feeling unwell following a car journey back to Belfast from Dublin having been to visit his girlfriend over the weekend. He has a headache and informs you that he had great difficulty concentrating on the final part of his trip. He does admit to having a 'big weekend' while in Dublin. On examination his pulse is bounding in character.

His various investigations are shown. The arterial blood gas was sampled with the patient breathing room air.

PasTest HOSPITAL

Na^+	140 mmol/l
K^+	4.2 mmol/l
Urea	4.8 mmol/l
Creatinine	76 µmol/l
Cl^-	105 mmol/l
HCO_3^-	23 mmol/l
pH	7.41
PaO_2	13.8 kPa
$PaCO_2$	4.3 kPa
HCO_3^-	24.3 mmol/l
Carboxyhaemoglobin	17%
Alcohol	nil
Urine – trace of cannabinoids	

Describe the abnormalities seen and explain the cause of this man's symptoms.

Answer 47

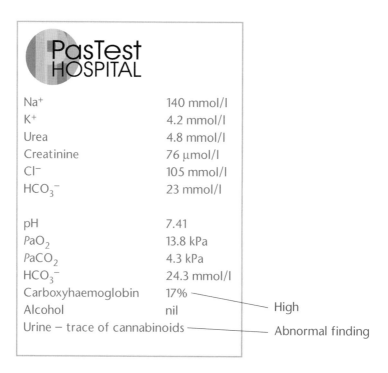

PasTest HOSPITAL

Na$^+$	140 mmol/l
K$^+$	4.2 mmol/l
Urea	4.8 mmol/l
Creatinine	76 μmol/l
Cl$^-$	105 mmol/l
HCO$_3$$^-$	23 mmol/l
pH	7.41
PaO$_2$	13.8 kPa
PaCO$_2$	4.3 kPa
HCO$_3$$^-$	24.3 mmol/l
Carboxyhaemoglobin	17% — High
Alcohol	nil
Urine – trace of cannabinoids	Abnormal finding

On first inspection, one might suspect that illicit drug use could provide the explanation for this patient's symptoms. However, another diagnosis may be more likely – carbon monoxide poisoning. This student developed symptoms following a car journey of several hours. Typically, students, the elderly and socially deprived people are most susceptible to exposure to carbon monoxide from poorly maintained fires and motor cars. Carbon monoxide poisoning can be diagnosed by measuring carboxyhaemoglobin in an arterial blood gas sample. This patient's carboxyhaemoglobin is elevated in keeping with the clinical suspicion. It is entirely appropriate that a urine drug screen has been performed, although the patient should be informed if this is being sent. A trace of cannabinoids suggests recent use of cannabis. This is, however, unlikely to be the explanation for this recent onset of symptoms.

Case 48

A 25-year-old shop assistant is brought to hospital by her colleague at 16:30 hours after she admitted to taking an overdose of paracetamol. She regrets the incident and is able to tell you clearly that she has taken one packet of 16 tablets during her lunch break between 12:00 and 12:30 hours. She feels fine and wishes to go home. No other medications or alcohol were taken. She has no health problems and is on no prescribed medications except the oral contraceptive pill. Blood tests taken on arrival at the hospital are shown.

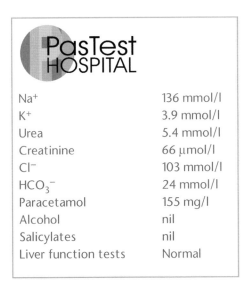

PasTest HOSPITAL

Na$^+$	136 mmol/l
K$^+$	3.9 mmol/l
Urea	5.4 mmol/l
Creatinine	66 µmol/l
Cl$^-$	103 mmol/l
HCO$_3^-$	24 mmol/l
Paracetamol	155 mg/l
Alcohol	nil
Salicylates	nil
Liver function tests	Normal

Would you treat this patient? Detail the logic for your decision.

Answer 48

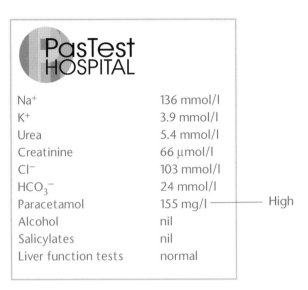

PasTest
HOSPITAL

Na^+	136 mmol/l
K^+	3.9 mmol/l
Urea	5.4 mmol/l
Creatinine	66 μmol/l
Cl^-	103 mmol/l
HCO_3^-	24 mmol/l
Paracetamol	155 mg/l ——— High
Alcohol	nil
Salicylates	nil
Liver function tests	normal

The three most important pieces of information to ascertain from a paracetamol overdose patient are:

- **How much has been taken?**
- **When was it taken?**
- **Does the patient have any factors to make them 'high risk'?**

Further questions to ascertain the psychiatric state and suicide risk are also clearly important.

In this case:

- **How much?**

16 tablets. Paracetamol tablets are 500 mg. Thus total dose = 16 x 500 mg = 8000 mg = 8 g.

- **Timing?**

4 h post ingestion.

- **Risk?**

No high-risk features from history

The 4 h level in this patient is 155 mg/l.

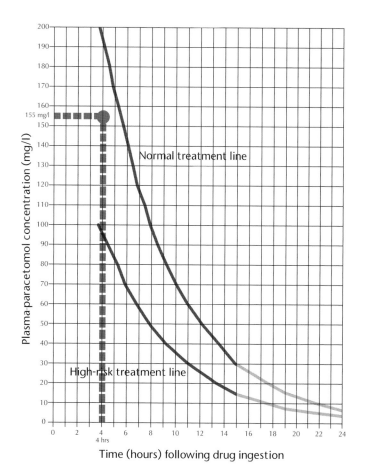

Time (hours) following drug ingestion

Using the graph illustrated earlier, one can interpret a paracetamol level of 155 mg/l at 4 h as not a high enough level to warrant treatment. Note, however, that if this patient was deemed to be 'high risk', treatment would have been necessary. The cut-off difference between the normal and high-risk groups at 4 h is substantial – 195 mg/l and 100 mg/l.

Case 49

A 33-year-old single mother attends A&E with her neighbour who found that she had taken an overdose when she came round to visit at tea time. The patient is a difficult historian but does indicate that she took about 30–50 tablets from the cupboard during the midday news. It is now 19:15 hours. The neighbour indicates that the woman has a history of epilepsy and she is on medication for this. Blood tests were taken on arrival.

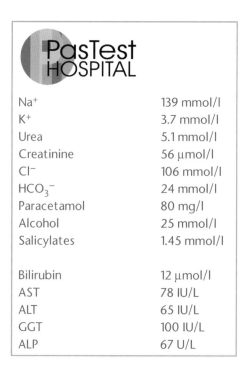

Na$^+$	139 mmol/l
K$^+$	3.7 mmol/l
Urea	5.1 mmol/l
Creatinine	56 μmol/l
Cl$^-$	106 mmol/l
HCO$_3^-$	24 mmol/l
Paracetamol	80 mg/l
Alcohol	25 mmol/l
Salicylates	1.45 mmol/l
Bilirubin	12 μmol/l
AST	78 IU/L
ALT	65 IU/L
GGT	100 IU/L
ALP	67 U/L

State what treatment this woman might need and justify your answer

Answer 49

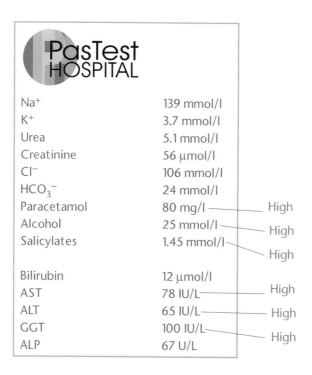

PasTest HOSPITAL		
Na⁺	139 mmol/l	
K⁺	3.7 mmol/l	
Urea	5.1 mmol/l	
Creatinine	56 µmol/l	
Cl⁻	106 mmol/l	
HCO₃⁻	24 mmol/l	
Paracetamol	80 mg/l	High
Alcohol	25 mmol/l	High
Salicylates	1.45 mmol/l	High
Bilirubin	12 µmol/l	
AST	78 IU/L	High
ALT	65 IU/L	High
GGT	100 IU/L	High
ALP	67 U/L	

This overdose case is more difficult, although perhaps more typical. The patient is only admitting to taking 'tablets', although the quantity, type and timing are more uncertain. At the time of presentation to hospital it is over 7 h since ingestion. To complicate matters further she is also on an unspecified anticonvulsant medication. This patient has taken alcohol with the tablets, has a raised paracetamol level and a mildly raised salicylate level. The patient also has mild impairment of her liver function tests.

On first glance 80 mg/l of paracetamol doesn't appear that remarkable. However, if the exact drug history cannot quickly be ascertained, one must assume that this patient is on hepatic enzyme-inducing antiepileptic medication. When this is transferred to the nomogram, one can see that a level of 80 mg/l is well above the treatment line in high-risk groups. Instigation of an infusion of NAC must commence immediately.

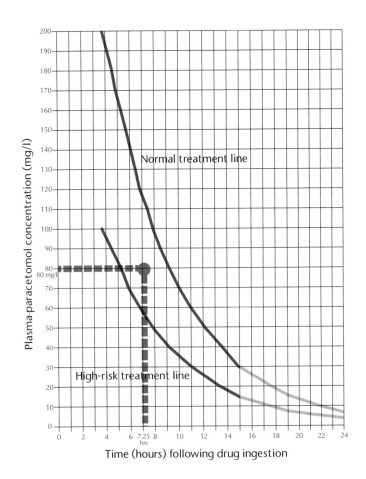

Time (hours) following drug ingestion

Case 50

A 41-year-old patient with bipolar disorder presents to A&E indicating that she has taken an overdose of her prescribed lithium. She is subdued and states that she had been feeling low at the time. Her examination is normal and she does not have any direct complaints. Blood tests are shown.

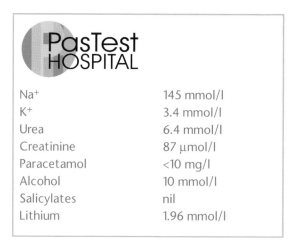

PasTest HOSPITAL	
Na$^+$	145 mmol/l
K$^+$	3.4 mmol/l
Urea	6.4 mmol/l
Creatinine	87 μmol/l
Paracetamol	<10 mg/l
Alcohol	10 mmol/l
Salicylates	nil
Lithium	1.96 mmol/l

Explain the treatment options in lithium overdose with specific reference to this patient.

Answer 50

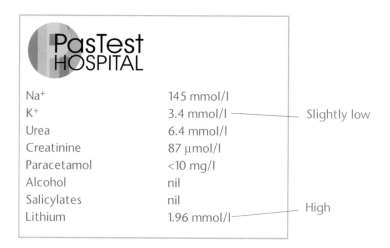

PasTest
HOSPITAL

Na+	145 mmol/l
K+	3.4 mmol/l —— Slightly low
Urea	6.4 mmol/l
Creatinine	87 µmol/l
Paracetamol	<10 mg/l
Alcohol	nil
Salicylates	nil
Lithium	1.96 mmol/l —— High

One must be particularly mindful in psychiatric patients of the accuracy of information conveyed and compliance with medication. Lithium is a commonly used drug in bipolar affective disorder, but has one major drawback – overdose. It has a narrow therapeutic ratio. Patients on long-term lithium can become unwell due to toxicity even without deliberate overdose. Overdoses of lithium can be fatal. The normal range is 0.4–1.5 mmol/l with levels above 2.0 mmol/l requiring treatment that may include haemodialysis. Levels between 1.5 and 2.0 mmol/l, as in this case, may require only fluid resuscitation and supportive treatment, along with temporary discontinuation of the drug.

PLEURAL AND PERITONEAL FLUID ANALYSIS

5

PLEURAL AND PERITONEAL FLUID ANALYSIS

In health, only a small volume of fluid surrounds the pleural lining of the lung. In various pathological states, excess fluid can accumulate forming a pleural effusion. When a significant volume has collected it may be detected on clinical examination or on a chest radiograph. Approximately 300 ml of fluid must be present before a pleural effusion is apparent on chest radiograph. Pleural fluid is not the only fluid that can collect within the pleural cavity. Blood in the pleural space is termed a haemothorax, lymph a chylothorax, and pus an empyema.

Analysis of this fluid may help determine the cause of the effusion. If significant volumes of fluid are removed there can also be symptomatic benefit to the patient. Fluid is collected by performing pleural aspiration ('a pleural tap') on the ward or, in difficult circumstances, in the radiology department under image guidance.

A number of key parameters are analysed routinely, with many additional tests being possible on request. The first fundamental point to establish is whether the effusion is an exudate or a transudate. This is determined principally by the protein content of the effusion. In the majority of cases, unilateral pleural effusions are exudates and bilateral effusions are transudates.

> **DON'T FORGET**
> Unilateral pleural effusions are nearly always exudates

Exudate ≥30 g/l of protein
Transudate <30 g/l of protein

The lactate dehydrogenase (LDH) level can also aid differentiation between exudates and transudates with a high level (greater than two-thirds of the upper limit of normal in blood) being in keeping with an exudate.

COMMON PARAMETERS ANALYSED IN PLEURAL FLUID	REASON FOR ANALYSIS
Total protein	Differentiate exudate and transudate
Lactate dehydrogenase (LDH)	Differentiate exudate and transudate
Microbiology (microscopy, cell count, gram stain and culture)	Identify an infection

ADDITIONAL PARAMETERS ANALYSED IN PLEURAL FLUID	INTERPRETATION
Glucose	Low in rheumatoid disease
Rheumatoid factor	High in rheumatoid disease
Amylase	High in pancreatitis
Ziehl–Nielson stain and culture	To diagnose tuberculosis
Cytology (large volume of fluid required)	To identify malignant cause of effusion
pH	Low in empyema

CAUSES OF A TRANSUDATE PLEURAL EFFUSION

Cardiac failure
Liver failure
Renal failure
Hypoalbuminaemia ('nutritional failure')
Hypothyroidism ('thyroid failure')

DON'T FORGET

Transudates are usually associated with FAILURE

CAUSES OF AN EXUDATE PLEURAL EFFUSION

Bronchial carcinoma
Pulmonary metastases
Mesothelioma
Pneumonia (parapneumonic effusion)
Pulmonary embolus/infarction
Tuberculosis
Connective tissue disease (eg rheumatoid disease)
Acute pancreatitis
Sarcoidosis

DON'T FORGET

An exudate exudes (pumps out) protein so the protein content is high

The colour of the fluid aspirated from a pleural effusion also gives useful information as to the potential cause.

COLOUR OF FLUID	DIAGNOSIS
Straw	Normal
Yellow	Infected
Blood stained	Traumatic, malignancy
Frank blood	Mesothelioma, trauma, other malignancy
Pus	Empyema

Case 51

A 36-year-old man is admitted with shortness of breath and a cough productive of green sputum. He is feverish and complains of left-sided pleuritic chest discomfort. He has led a perfectly healthy life to date. He is a smoker of 10 pack-years. On examination a pleural effusion is noted on the left side to the mid-zone. This finding is confirmed on chest radiograph.

The effusion is aspirated at ward level and sent for analysis.

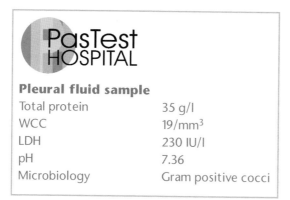

PasTest
HOSPITAL

Pleural fluid sample

Total protein	35 g/l
WCC	19/mm³
LDH	230 IU/l
pH	7.36
Microbiology	Gram positive cocci

Describe the findings and the likely cause of the pleural effusion.

Answer 51

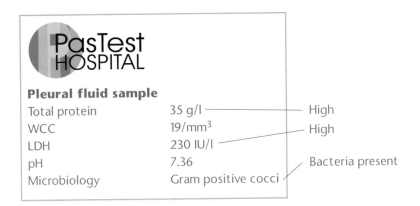

PasTest HOSPITAL

Pleural fluid sample

Total protein	35 g/l	High
WCC	19/mm³	High
LDH	230 IU/l	
pH	7.36	Bacteria present
Microbiology	Gram positive cocci	

This patient has symptoms suggestive of a bacterial pneumonia. He is otherwise healthy and there is little to suspect an underlying sinister or chronic disease. A proportion of bacterial pneumonias will present with a pleural effusion. Pleural fluid is produced in excess in reaction to the local irritation of the pleura from the surrounding infection.

The findings from the simple pleural fluid analysis are in keeping with this clinical suspicion. It is an exudate (total protein > 30 g/l) and the lactate dehydrogenase level is high. Further confirmation of a bacterial cause is noted with the finding of Gram-positive cocci. This would most likely represent an infection with *Streptococcus pneumoniae*.

This patient has a parapneumonic pleural effusion. Treatment consists of antibiotics for the pneumonia, with the effusion expected to resolve over several weeks. The patient should have a repeat chest radiograph 6 weeks after treatment to ensure resolution of the effusion. If the patient's condition were to deteriorate one would have to consider the development of an empyema (pus collection in the pleural space).

Case 52

A 65-year-old retired headmaster presents with progressive shortness of breath and swelling of the feet. Nine years ago he sustained an anterior myocardial infarction and has had subsequent problems with angina requiring coronary artery stenting. He also suffers from hypertension and gout. Following a recent flare of gout his GP prescribed a short course of ibuprofen. Examination reveals pitting oedema to the mid-calves bilaterally and a jugular venous pulse (JVP) raised by 3 cm H_2O. The bases of both lungs are dull to percussion. Breath sounds are reduced and vocal resonance is decreased over these areas.

After some initial treatment these examination findings remain and a decision is made to carry out pleural aspiration: 30 ml was aspirated from the right hemithorax and sent for analysis.

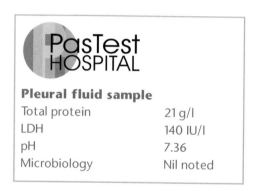

PasTest HOSPITAL

Pleural fluid sample

Total protein	21 g/l
LDH	140 IU/l
pH	7.36
Microbiology	Nil noted

Describe the findings and likely cause.

Answer 52

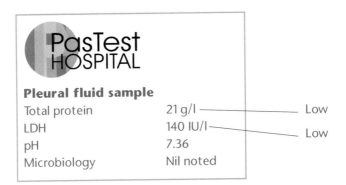

Pleural fluid sample

Total protein	21 g/l	Low
LDH	140 IU/l	Low
pH	7.36	
Microbiology	Nil noted	

The clinical features of this patient suggest a diagnosis of congestive cardiac failure (CCF). The prescription of a non-steroidal anti-inflammatory drug (NSAID) for acute gout has caused fluid retention leading to worsening of underlying cardiac failure. The effusions are bilateral, which suggests that they are likely to be transudative. The pleural fluid sample confirms this suspicion with a total protein content of only 21 g/l and an LDH of 140 IU/l. Of all the causes of transudate pleural effusions, cardiac failure best fits in this case.

Case 53

As the medical SHO you are asked by your surgical colleagues to see a 45-year-old overweight housewife . She was admitted with abdominal pain 2 days ago and an ultrasound scan of the abdomen showed gallstones with extra hepatic bile duct dilatation. Bowel gas obscured visualisation of the pancreas. Your opinion is sought as the patient is short of breath and complains of left-sided pleuritic chest discomfort. On examination you detect a left-sided pleural effusion which is confirmed on chest radiograph. You decide to perform a diagnostic pleural aspiration.

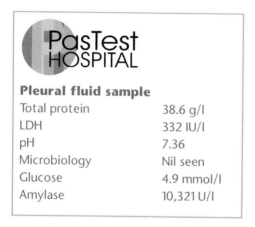

PasTest HOSPITAL

Pleural fluid sample

Total protein	38.6 g/l
LDH	332 IU/l
pH	7.36
Microbiology	Nil seen
Glucose	4.9 mmol/l
Amylase	10,321 U/l

What is your interpretation of this result?

Answer 53

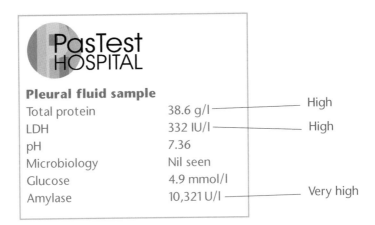

PasTest HOSPITAL

Pleural fluid sample

Total protein	38.6 g/l	High
LDH	332 IU/l	High
pH	7.36	
Microbiology	Nil seen	
Glucose	4.9 mmol/l	
Amylase	10,321 U/l	Very high

Pleural effusions can be found in acute pancreatitis. It is most typical for this to be unilateral; however, bilateral effusions are recognised. The key to diagnosis is the amylase level within the aspirated fluid.

Case 54

A 33-year-old secretary presents with malaise, joint discomfort and by her own admission generally feeling 'out of sorts'. She was diagnosed with Graves' disease 3 years ago and has been rendered euthyroid (normal thyroid function). She has also suffered from coeliac disease since her teens. She has no respiratory complaints. As part of her investigative work-up a chest radiograph is taken, which to the medical team's surprise shows a right-sided pleural effusion of moderate size.

Pleural aspiration is performed.

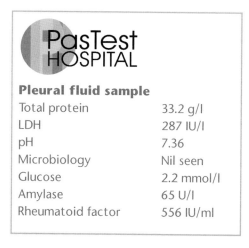

PasTest HOSPITAL

Pleural fluid sample

Total protein	33.2 g/l
LDH	287 IU/l
pH	7.36
Microbiology	Nil seen
Glucose	2.2 mmol/l
Amylase	65 U/l
Rheumatoid factor	556 IU/ml

What is the cause of her effusion?

Answer 54

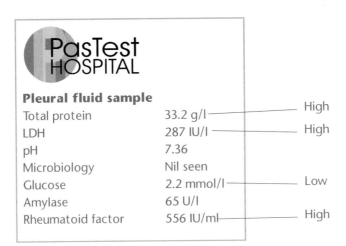

Pleural fluid sample

Total protein	33.2 g/l	High
LDH	287 IU/l	High
pH	7.36	
Microbiology	Nil seen	
Glucose	2.2 mmol/l	Low
Amylase	65 U/l	
Rheumatoid factor	556 IU/ml	High

Pleural effusion is an uncommon but well-documented finding in rheumatoid disease. This is a systemic disease and a number of manifestations occur in the chest. Among these are: pleural effusion, pulmonary nodules, interstitial fibrosis, pleural thickening and bronchiolitis obliterans. This patient has a number of autoimmune diseases so it would not be unreasonable for her to be diagnosed with rheumatoid disease. The pleural effusion is an exudate. The rheumatoid factor level is hugely elevated at 556 IU/ml. In addition the glucose is low at 2.2 mmol/l in the effusion, further supporting the diagnosis.

Peritoneal fluid analysis

In health, peritoneal fluid is present only in small volumes. In illness it may collect in vast quantities, in which case it should be detected on clinical examination. Smaller volumes may be detected on imaging. An abnormal collection of peritoneal fluid is termed ascites.

Paracentesis (often termed 'peritoneal tap') may be undertaken for diagnostic purposes. Alternatively, large volumes of fluid can be removed to provide symptomatic benefit to the patient.

Analysis of peritoneal fluid has two main purposes:

- To characterise the disease causing ascites
- To detect infection.

The parameters shown in the box may be analysed. Those marked with an asterisk should be requested only when clinically indicated.

PARAMETER	PURPOSE
WCC (including differential)	To detect peritonitis ; neutrophils ↑ c̄ SBP
Total protein content	To distinguish exudates and transudates. To calculate the serum–ascites albumin gradient
Microscopy including Gram stain	To visualise bacteria
Culture	To identify bacteria
Glucose*	Low in malignant ascites
Cytology*	To detect malignant cells
Amylase*	Raised in ascites associated with pancreatitis

Characterising the disease causing ascites

The most common cause of ascites by far is portal hypertension secondary to liver cirrhosis. However, there are a great many other causes. It is important to be able to distinguish between these.

In a method analogous to pleural fluid analysis, the causes of ascites can be divided into whether they cause an exudate or a transudate. The total protein content is used to differentiate between the two, with a cut-off level of 25 g/l.

Exudate ≥ 25 g/l of protein
Transudate < 25 g/l of protein

CAUSES OF TRANSUDATE ASCITES

Cirrhosis
Cardiac failure
Hypoalbuminaemia
Nephrotic syndrome

CAUSES OF EXUDATE ASCITES

Intraperitoneal infection including tuberculosis
Intraperitoneal malignancy (primary or secondary)
Pancreatitis
Hypothyroidism
Chylous ascites

A more reliable method of characterising peritoneal fluid involves comparing the albumin content in the ascites with that in the blood. In doing so, the serum–ascites albumin gradient (SAAG) can be calculated.

> **Serum–ascites albumin gradient**
> **SAAG (g/l) = Serum albumin (g/l) – Ascites albumin (g/l)**

If the SAAG is ≥11 g/l, one can say that the patient is very likely to have portal hypertension. Bear in mind, however, that he or she may have portal hypertension plus another cause of ascites.

Detecting infection

The WCC of the ascites is increased in peritonitis. In most patients with ascites associated with cirrhosis, peritonitis is a primary problem, and is termed *spontaneous bacterial peritonitis* (SBP). Occasionally another cause of peritonitis, such as a subphrenic abscess or perforated bowel, can be mistaken for SBP.

The diagnosis of SBP can be made when bacteria are identified after culturing ascitic fluid. However, this process takes some time, so the ascites' WCC is usually used to guide treatment. This result should be available within a matter of hours. An ascites neutrophil count ≥250 cells/mm^3 (0.25 x 10^9/l) is in keeping with SBP. If the clinical setting fits with this diagnosis, treatment with an appropriate antibiotic should be commenced.

> **DON'T FORGET**
> Ascites neutrophil count of ≥250 cells/mm^3 is in keeping with SBP

An alternative cause for peritonitis (eg perforated bowel) should be suspected when multiple organisms are seen on Gram staining.

Case 55

A 42-year-old salesman with established alcoholic liver cirrhosis is a known patient to the ward. He has been admitted on multiple previous occasions and continues to drink heavily. On this admission he is a little confused and tremulous. On examination, ascites is present along with small bilateral pleural effusions. His abdomen is mildly tender throughout. Bowel sounds are present.

The on-call SHO performs a diagnostic peritoneal aspiration on the admissions ward. One hour later, the laboratory technician phones with the report below.

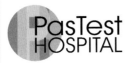

Analysis of peritoneal fluid

WCC	322 cells/mm^3 – predominantly neutrophils
Albumin	16 g/l
Amylase	92 U/l
Microscopy	Gram-negative cocci seen on Gram stain

His blood albumin level is 29 g/l.

What is the diagnosis, and how should the patient be treated?

Answer 55

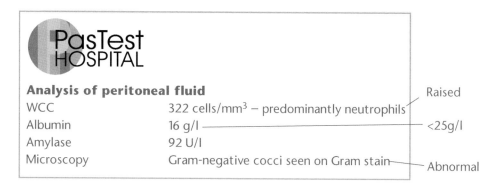

PasTest HOSPITAL

Analysis of peritoneal fluid		
WCC	322 cells/mm³ – predominantly neutrophils	Raised
Albumin	16 g/l	<25g/l
Amylase	92 U/l	
Microscopy	Gram-negative cocci seen on Gram stain	Abnormal

His ascites white cell count shows a neutrophilia, with more than 250 cells/mm³.

The albumin content is less than 25 g/l indicating a transudate.

The SAAG is 13 g/l (29 g/l – 16 g/l). This is in keeping with portal hypertension.

Gram staining shows the most typical finding in SBP – Gram-negative cocci. In time, one might expect culture to yield *Escherichia coli* or *Klebsiella* species.

This man has spontaneous bacterial peritonitis, on a background of hepatic cirrhosis caused by alcohol. His clinical features are typical with general abdominal discomfort, often accompanied by pyrexia. This infection has also made him mildly encephalopathic, hence the confusion.

In a patient with a history of alcohol dependency, abdominal distension and pain, pancreatitis is a further differential diagnosis. However, this would cause an exudate, and one would expect the amylase level to be raised significantly.

Case 56

A frail 88-year-old nursing home resident is brought to hospital because of abdominal pain. Her nurse is also concerned regarding the progressive increase in her abdominal girth over the past 6 weeks. She has a history of vascular dementia. On examination there is a grossly distended abdomen, with shifting dullness and a fluid thrill. A CT scan of the abdomen and pelvis demonstrated a massive mixed solid-cystic lesion and gross ascites within the pelvis.

Peritoneal aspiration was performed for diagnostic purposes and symptomatic benefit: 9500 ml was drained and sent for analysis. The results are shown.

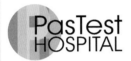

PasTest HOSPITAL

Analysis of peritoneal fluid

WCC	25 cells/mm^3 – mixed leukocytes
Albumin	28 g/l
Microscopy	No organisms seen
Cytology	Tumour cells seen – in keeping with adenocarcinoma

Her blood albumin level is 29 g/l.

Provide a diagnosis and explain your reasoning.

Answer 56

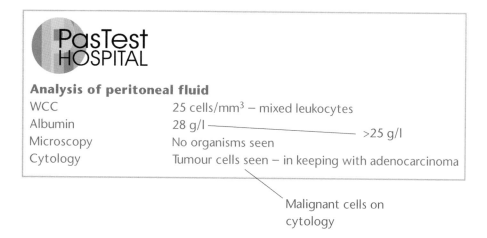

PasTest
HOSPITAL

Analysis of peritoneal fluid

WCC	25 cells/mm³ – mixed leukocytes
Albumin	28 g/l ——————————————— >25 g/l
Microscopy	No organisms seen
Cytology	Tumour cells seen – in keeping with adenocarcinoma

Malignant cells on
cytology

The WCC is not significantly raised.

The albumin level is greater than 25 g/l, indicating an exudate.

The SAAG is 1 g/l (29 g/l – 28 g/l) indicating a low probability of portal hypertension.

The diagnosis is seen on cytology.

This patient has an advanced intraperitoneal malignancy. The specific primary origin is unknown. The cells present may originate from a primary intra-peritoneal malignancy or be due to intraperitoneal metastatic disease. A large volume of ascites in an elderly patient without known liver disease should always arouse the suspicion of malignancy. The CT findings are in keeping with a primary pelvic malignancy.

Case 57

A 36-year-old banker attends A&E complaining of recurrent bouts of intense abdominal discomfort. He has been reluctant to present previously for fear of admission. He admits to being a heavy drinker, but his family and colleagues are not aware of his problem. On examination there is distension of the abdomen with ascites present, tenderness in the upper abdomen and a faint upper midline incision.

You are concerned about his level of abdominal pain. He agrees to peritoneal aspiration, but does not wish to be admitted.

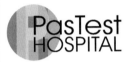

Analysis of peritoneal fluid

WCC	147 cells/mm^3 – predominantly neutrophils
Albumin	29 g/l
Amylase	894 U/l
Microscopy	No organisms seen

The patient's blood albumin level is 32 g/l.

Give a diagnosis and list useful further investigations.

Answer 57

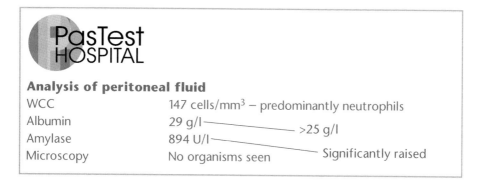

PasTest
HOSPITAL

Analysis of peritoneal fluid

WCC	147 cells/mm³ – predominantly neutrophils
Albumin	29 g/l ——————— >25 g/l
Amylase	894 U/l ——
Microscopy	No organisms seen ——— Significantly raised

The ascites is an exudate, and there is no evidence of infection.

The SAAG is 3 g/l (32 g/l – 29 g/l), indicating a low probability of portal hypertension.

The amylase is hugely elevated at 894 U/l, in keeping with acute pancreatitis.

Every effort should be made to persuade this man of the need to stay in hospital for further investigation and treatment of his pancreatitis.

MICROBIOLOGY

6

MICROBIOLOGY

Micro-organisms feature in the clinical problems of many patients. Bacteria predominate in most clinical settings.

Bodily fluids and swabs from surface sites may be collected and sent for microbiological analysis. Blood, urine and sputum are the most commonly analysed. Samples may be examined directly by light microscopy to provide a quick result. Generally, however, more useful information is obtained when samples are cultured. This process takes several days in most circumstances. Prolonged culture (ie weeks) is required when testing for the presence of mycobacteria.

The basic stain used with light microscopy is haematoxylin and eosin (H&E). Gram-positive organisms stain blue. Gram-negative organisms stain pink.

Bacteria may be subdivided further on the basis of their shape. Rod-shaped bacteria are termed bacilli. Spherical bacteria are termed cocci.

A reasonable 'best guess' as to the identity of a bacterium may be made after studying the Gram-staining characteristics and shape by microscopy. Bacteria may be classified further into either aerobic or anaerobic based on their growth requirements when being cultured. Common examples are shown in the box below.

EXAMPLES OF COMMON ORGANISMS		
Aerobes	Gram-positive cocci	Staphylococcus aureus Streptococcus pyogenes Streptococcus pneumoniae Enterococcus faecalis
	Gram-positive bacilli	Listeria monocytogenes Bacillus anthracis
	Gram-negative cocci	Moraxella catarrhalis Neisseria meningitidis
	Gram-negative bacilli	Escherichia coli Pseudomonas aeruginosa
Anaerobes	Cocci	Peptococci Peptostreptococci
	Bacilli	Bacteroides fragilis Clostridium difficile

An important and common Gram-positive coccus is *Staphylococcus aureus*. This bacterium is divided on the basis of its coagulase enzyme activity into coagulase positive or negative.

Streptococci are classified by their action on erythrocytes into alpha- and beta- haemolytic types.

Once a micro-organism is identified, its sensitivity to a batch of suitable common antibiotics is tested at the time of culturing. There are three typical outcomes to antibiotic testing:

- Sensitive (S)

- Intermediately sensitive (I)

- Resistant (R).

A typical culture and sensitivity report would be as follows:

PasTest
HOSPITAL

Urine culture

> 10^5 organisms/ml *Proteus* species

Co-amoxiclav	R
Ampicillin	S
Ciprofloxacin	S
Cefotaxime	S
Nitrofurantoin	I
Tazocin	S
Trimethoprim	R
Cephalexin	S

In the example, the most appropriate antibiotics to prescribe are shown as sensitive (S).

A small number of antibiotics require monitoring of the serum levels, the commonest being the aminoglycoside gentamicin. Others include teicoplanin and vancomycin. The level should be checked after 'loading' of the drug and at regular intervals during the treatment course.

It should always be considered that a positive culture result might merely represent contamination. Contamination is particularly common in blood and urine specimens, and highlights the importance of careful technique when taking such samples. A common finding on a contaminated blood culture sample is the finding of coagulase-negative staphylococci. This finding is often due to *Staphylococcus epidermidis* – a bacterium that is part of the normal skin flora.

DON'T FORGET
Always consider the possibility of sample contamination

Hospital-acquired (nosocomial) infections represent a significant morbidity and mortality. Special mention should be given to methicillin-resistant *Staphylococcus aureus* (MRSA) and *Clostridium difficile*. These conditions impose a significant burden on infection control teams.

One should be aware of opportunistic micro-organisms. These are a group of micro-organisms that occur most commonly in immunosuppressed patients, and include *Pneumocystis carinii* and *Mycobacterium avium intracellulare*.

Interpretation of microbiological data is found within Chapter 16, Complete Clinical Cases.

Urinalysis

The urine, ideally a mid-stream sample, may be analysed quickly and easily at a ward level. A range of parameters can be checked with a simple reagent strip. Each reagent undergoes a colour change which varies depending on the amount of a particular substance that is present.

The range of possible urinalysis results is shown in the table below.

Glucose	Neg	Trace	+	++	+++	++++	
Bilirubin	Neg	+	++	+++			
Ketones	Neg	Trace	+	++	+++	++++	
Specific gravity	1.000	1.005	1.010	1.015	1.020	1.025	1.030
Blood	Neg	Trace (non-haem-olysed)	++ (non-haem-olysed)	Trace (haem-olysed)	+ (haem-olysed)	++ (haem-olysed)	+++ (haem-olysed)
pH	5.0	6.0	6.5	7.0	7.5	8.0	8.5
Protein	Neg	Trace	+	++	+++	++++	
Urobilinogen (mg/dl)	0.2	1	2	4	≥8		
Nitrite	Neg	Pos					
Leukocytes	Neg	Trace	+	++	+++		

Possible results on urinalysis

Nitrites and leukocytes are commonly positive in the setting of a urinary tract infection.

NEUROLOGICAL
INVESTIGATIONS

7

NEUROLOGICAL INVESTIGATIONS

There are three main groups of tests used to investigate neurological disease. Cerebrospinal fluid analysis and neurophysiological investigations are dealt with in this chapter. Imaging is touched upon in Chapter 9. It is the combination of findings from these tests, rather than one in isolation, that frequently enables a diagnosis to be made.

Cerebrospinal fluid analysis

Cerebrospinal fluid (CSF) is obtained by performing a lumbar puncture. A number of parameters are checked during routine analysis. More specialist tests are undertaken only in certain circumstances (see boxes).

A methodical approach to the interpretation of results is helpful.

COMPONENTS OF A ROUTINE CSF ANALYSIS	
Appearance	Glucose
Presence of organisms	White cell count
(Gram stain + culture)	(+ differential if raised)
Total protein	Red cell count

OTHER TESTS	ASSOCIATED WITH
Xanthochromia	Subarachnoid haemorrhage
Oligoclonal bands	Multiple sclerosis
Herpes simplex/zoster serology	Herpes meningitis/encephalitis
Neuropathology	CNS tumours
Protein 14-3-3	Creutzfeldt–Jakob disease
Lyme disease serology (*Borrelia burgdorferi*)	Lyme disease
Angiotensin-converting enzyme	Neurosarcoidosis

It is essential when performing a lumbar puncture to ensure that a blood sample is taken simultaneously and analysed for plasma glucose as well as total protein content. This is to enable the calculation of a CSF:plasma ratio. This helps distinguish between different infectious causes of meningitis.

DON'T FORGET

Always remember to take a concurrent blood sample for protein and glucose

The appearance of the CSF is also helpful. It should be clear. In bacterial meningitis it appears cloudy and in subarachnoid haemorrhage (SAH) it may be bloody.

CSF is often analysed for the presence of xanthochromia when an SAH is suspected. The test is performed because a proportion of SAHs will not be seen on a CT scan of the brain. The timing of this sample in relation to the onset of headache is important, in that lumbar puncture should be carried out at least 12 h after the onset of the headache. However, delaying lumbar puncture for too long is not advised, since, the longer the lumbar puncture is delayed, the lower the chance of detecting xanthochromia.

DON'T FORGET

Timing of a xanthochromia sample is vital

Case 58

A 19-year-old university student complains of a headache of 8 h duration accompanied by a dislike for lights. She has vomited twice. She is sweaty to touch. No rash is apparent. The A&E officer was concerned enough to request a CT scan of the brain which was reported as normal. She proceeds to lumbar puncture. The CSF pressure was normal at the time of lumbar puncture.

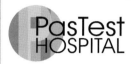

PasTest
HOSPITAL

Appearance	Cloudy. No organisms seen
WCC	228/mm^3 (predominantly neutrophils)
Red cell count	4/mm^3
Glucose	2.1 mmol/l
Total protein	0.96 g/l
Plasma glucose	5.9 mmol/l
Plasma total protein	0.45 g/l

Describe the CSF, and state the most likely diagnosis.

Answer 58

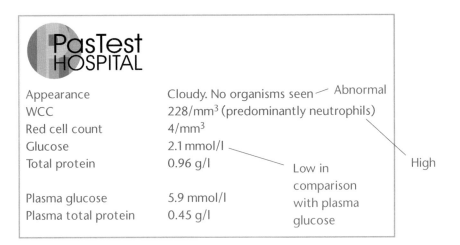

PasTest
HOSPITAL

Appearance	Cloudy. No organisms seen — Abnormal
WCC	228/mm³ (predominantly neutrophils)
Red cell count	4/mm³
Glucose	2.1 mmol/l
Total protein	0.96 g/l
Plasma glucose	5.9 mmol/l
Plasma total protein	0.45 g/l

Low in comparison with plasma glucose

High

Several features in the history should set off alarm bells for bacterial meningitis. The patient is young and in an institutional environment, and has an acute headache with photophobia. In addition, the CSF is cloudy with a raised WCC and a low CSF:plasma glucose ratio.

Three important points can be learned from this case:

1. If the leukocyte count is raised, analysis of the differential leukocyte count will help in distinguishing the cause.

2. A patient may have bacterial meningitis without any organisms being seen on microscopy. Don't be put off by this.

3. In bacterial meningitis, CT imaging of the brain can be normal even when the CSF is highly abnormal.

This patient has bacterial meningitis and requires immediate treatment with intravenous antibiotics. Benzylpenicillin or cefotaxime is the antibiotic of choice in most cases if the patient is not allergic.

THE CLASSIC CSF FINDINGS IN BACTERIAL MENINGITIS:	
A cloudy appearance	Raised (but only mild–moderate)
Organisms seen in CSF	total protein
Raised WCC	Significantly reduced CSF glucose
(with >95% neutrophils)	Reduced CSF:plasma glucose ratio
Red cell count (RCC) normal	(to less than two-thirds)

Case 59

A 21-year-old soldier complains of a headache for the past 2 days and a dislike for the light. He is feverish. He has recently returned from deployment in Germany. Examination did not reveal any focal neurological signs or signs suggestive of raised intracranial pressure. The CSF opening pressure at the time of lumbar puncture was normal (17 mmH$_2$O). Lumbar puncture is performed, and the following result obtained.

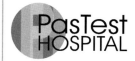

PasTest
HOSPITAL

Appearance	Clear. No organisms seen
WCC	101/mm^3 (>95% lymphocytes)
RCC	9/mm^3
Glucose	3.9 mmol/l
Total protein	1.4 g/l
Plasma glucose	5.8 mmol/l
Plasma total protein	0.45 g/l

Interpret this CSF sample and give a differential diagnosis of the cause.

Answer 59

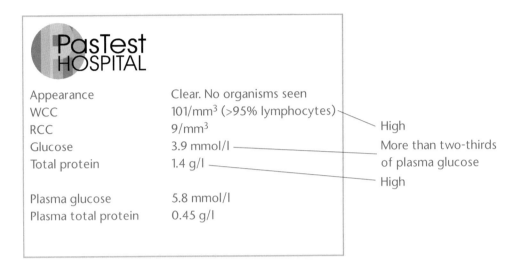

PasTest
HOSPITAL

Appearance	Clear. No organisms seen
WCC	101/mm³ (>95% lymphocytes)
RCC	9/mm³
Glucose	3.9 mmol/l
Total protein	1.4 g/l
Plasma glucose	5.8 mmol/l
Plasma total protein	0.45 g/l

High

More than two-thirds
of plasma glucose

High

This history is not dissimilar to Case 58. However, the CSF analysis is significantly different. The WCC is raised – although less so than in the example of bacterial meningitis. The differential WCC is also different – lymphocytes being the predominant cell type here. The plasma glucose is a little less than normal, as is the CSF:plasma glucose ratio. Total protein is elevated – but only marginally. In summary many of the parameters are abnormal, but not markedly so.

CAUSES OF LYMPHOCYTE-PREDOMINANT LEUKOCYTOSIS IN CSF

Viral meningitis	Tuberculous meningitis
Mumps meningoencephalitis	Partially treated bacterial meningitis

The most common cause for these findings is viral meningitis – the virus itself may never be identified. Polymerase chain reaction analysis of CSF can be performed to test for a number of viruses, including herpes simplex. The treatment and outcome of viral meningitis are markedly different to those of partially treated bacterial meningitis, and if any diagnostic doubt exists treatment should continue for bacterial meningitis. The reason for partial treatment may have been the commencement of an antibiotic by a GP.

Case 60

A 39-year-old man is admitted to the neurology ward following a short illness. He is unable to move his legs. He was previously well, although he did have a short bout of diarrhoea a week ago following his return from holiday in Turkey.

Lumbar puncture was performed. The CSF opening pressure at the time of lumbar puncture was 18 mmH$_2$O.

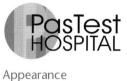

Appearance	Clear. No organisms seen
WCC	5/mm^3
RCC	2/mm^3
Glucose	3.6 mmol/l
Total protein	2.1 g/l
Plasma glucose	4.7 mmol/l
Plasma total protein	0.45 g/l

1. **What are the significant findings and what condition could cause this appearance?**

2. **What other test might help in coming to a diagnosis?**

Answer 60

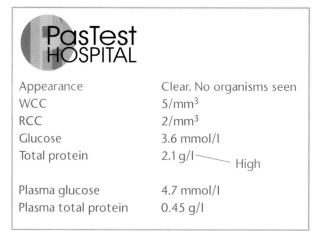

PasTest HOSPITAL

Appearance	Clear. No organisms seen
WCC	5/mm^3
RCC	2/mm^3
Glucose	3.6 mmol/l
Total protein	2.1 g/l —— High
Plasma glucose	4.7 mmol/l
Plasma total protein	0.45 g/l

1. The history is short and the symptoms significant. However, the only abnormality on the CSF sample is the elevated level of protein within the CSF. The plasma total protein is normal. The CSF protein is raised to a greater degree than one would usually expect for a viral or bacterial meningitis/encephalitis. Note that the WCC and the CSF:plasma glucose ratio are also not in keeping with an infective pathology. The differential diagnosis is therefore of a high CSF protein.

CAUSES OF RAISED CSF PROTEIN ·	
Mild–moderate	**High**
Viral meningitis	Guillain–Barré syndrome
Bacterial meningitis	Spinal block
Tuberculous meningitis	
Fungal meningitis	
Cerebral abscess	
Neoplastic meningitis	
Connective tissue disease	

When interpreted in the context of the history of leg weakness following an episode of infectious diarrhoea, the diagnosis is most likely to be Guillain–Barré syndrome (an acute inflammatory polyneuropathy).

2. Nerve conduction studies (NCS) would help diagnosis (see Neurophysiological investigations on page 199 for further details).

Case 61

A 29-year-old bank clerk has become known to local neurologists over the past year following several presentations to both the hospital and the outpatient clinic with a variable constellation of neurological symptoms. Initially a complaint of numbness over the lateral aspect of the left leg was mentioned. This resolved. Of late, she has had an episode of loss of vision in the right eye lasting 4 weeks. Examination reveals global hyper-reflexia and a mild cerebellar gait.

The patient attends the ward for a series of tests including lumbar puncture. The CSF opening pressure was 17 mmH$_2$O.

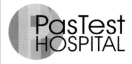
PasTest
HOSPITAL

Appearance	Clear. No organisms seen
WCC	11/mm^3
RCC	1/mm^3
Glucose	3.9 mmol/l
Total protein	0.46 g/l
Oligoclonal bands	Present
ACE level	Normal

A blood sample was taken at the same time:

Plasma glucose	5.1 mmol/l
Plasma total protein	0.46 g/l
Oligoclonal bands	Absent

What is the likely diagnosis?

Answer 61

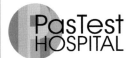

Appearance   Clear. No organisms seen
WCC   11/mm³
RCC   1/mm³
Glucose   3.9 mmol/l
Total protein   0.46 g/l
Oligoclonal bands   Present
ACE level   Normal   Abnormal

A blood sample was taken at the same time:
Plasma glucose   5.1 mmol/l
Plasma total protein   0.46 g/l

Oligoclonal bands   Absent

This CSF sample shows essentially normal values for all the common indices. Additional analyses have been performed, including oligoclonal bands which are present.

These bands represent immunoglobulin G (IgG). The presence of this has been noted in a number of conditions – it is therefore of poor specificity in isolation. However, it is found in over 80% of patients with multiple sclerosis (MS). MS is the most common cause for its presence on CSF analysis. It is a supportive feature rather than a diagnostic feature of the disease, since MS is a clinical diagnosis defined as 'two episodes of neurological deficit disseminated in time and place'.

CAUSES OF OLIGOCLONAL BANDS IN CSF

Multiple sclerosis
Subacute sclerosing panencephalitis
Guillain–Barré syndrome
Neurosyphilis
Lyme disease
Neurosarcoidosis

Neurophysiological investigations

Neurophysiology is a specialist domain within neurology. Only a brief understanding of the common investigations is necessary for an undergraduate. Likewise, knowledge of the key findings in classic conditions will suffice. It is unlikely that one would be expected to interpret neurophysiological investigations.

The main investigations to be aware of are nerve conduction studies and electromyography. Visually evoked responses and electroencephalography are further aids to diagnosis.

NEUROPHYSIOLOGICAL INVESTIGATIONS

Nerve conduction studies
Electromyography
Visually evoked responses
Electroencephalography

Nerve conduction studies (NCSs)

Nerve conduction studies measure how well individual nerves transmit electrical signals. The nerve of interest is stimulated, usually electrically, with surface electrodes placed on the skin. One electrode stimulates the nerve and the resulting electrical activity is recorded by the other electrodes. The distance between electrodes and the time taken for electrical impulses to travel between electrodes are used to calculate the nerve conduction velocity.

The commonest reason for NCSs to be requested is for suspected carpal tunnel syndrome. In this condition, the median nerve is entrapped within the confines of the carpal tunnel.

Electromyography (EMG)

Surface or needle electrodes are used to detect muscle action potentials following controlled electrical stimulation. The electrical stimulation provokes action potentials within the nerves which in turn stimulate a magnified response in muscles.

EMG may be modified for some indications. The most important to know is single-fibre EMG and EMG with repetitive stimulation used when myasthenia gravis is clinically suspected.

Visually evoked responses (VERs)

In this test, the eye is stimulated in order to evoke a response within the optic nerve. It is performed by placing a series of electrodes over the scalp in the occipital area whilst asking the patient to observe a series of visual patterns. The response of the optic nerve is recorded via the electrodes. Two indices are noted:

- The speed of response of the nerve (termed P100 latencies)

- The height of the waveform obtained.

This test is usually performed in patients in whom multiple sclerosis is suspected. In multiple sclerosis, the waveform will be preserved, but the speed of response will be delayed because of optic nerve demyelination.

Electroencephalography (EEG)

EEG is the recording of electrical activity from the brain using a series of scalp electrodes. Usually, recordings over a period of several minutes are taken. Broadly speaking, EEG can be used to diagnose epilepsy and diffuse brain disease. In epilepsy, it is most valuable if a recording takes place during a seizure since it is not unusual to obtain a normal recording between seizures.

In difficult cases, EEG recording can take place over several hours or days in a supervised room in hospital with video recording. EEG may also be invaluable in diagnosing non-convulsive status epilepticus and distinguishing true seizures from pseudoseizures. In non-convulsive status epilepticus, a patient is having ongoing seizures, despite these not manifesting themselves clinically. Prompt diagnosis by EEG may prevent a permanent neurological deficit.

Classic neurophysiological disease associations

TEST	RESULT	DISEASE
EEG	Spike and wave	Primary generalised epilepsy
EEG	Periodic complexes	Creutzfeldt–Jakob disease
EMG	Short polyphasic motor potentials Sometimes spontaneous fibrillation and high frequency repetitive discharges	Polymyositis
EMG (single fibre)	Fatiguability following repetitive stimulation	Myasthenia gravis
EMG	Repetitive single motor unit potentials all low amplitude. Short duration polyphasic motor unit potentials	Myotonic dystrophy
EMG	Spontaneous fibrillations	Motor neuron disease
NCS	Delay in conduction of median nerve	Carpal tunnel syndrome (entrapment neuropathy)
VERs	Delayed P100 latencies, without amplitude loss.	Multiple sclerosis

IMMUNOLOGY

8

IMMUNOLOGY

Interpretation of autoantibodies is often difficult. This is because of the degree of overlap in the presence of antibodies between various disease states. For example, rheumatoid factor can be found in well over a dozen diseases. Furthermore, certain autoantibodies may be found in healthy people, and the absence of an autoantibody may not rule out a particular disease. Therefore, always bear in mind that the presence of an autoantibody does not necessarily mean that a patient has a particular disease.

DON'T FORGET
A disease may be present without the typical autoantibody profile

For the purpose of undergraduate examinations, the classic autoantibody associations will be tested. These are listed in the box below. Those tested commonly in examinations are in bold type.

DISEASE	AUTOANTIBODIES
Addison's disease	Anti-21-hydroxylase
Anti-phospholipid syndrome	**Anti-cardiolipin** **Lupus anticoagulant antibodies**
Autoimmune haemolytic anaemia	**Red blood cell autoantibodies** (this disease can be classified into warm and cold, depending on the temperature at which the antibodies best attach to red cells)
Autoimmune hepatitis	**Anti-nuclear** **Anti-smooth muscle** **Anti-liver/kidney microsomal-I** Myeloperoxidase anti-nuclear cytoplasmic antibody (MPO-ANCA), also called perinuclear ANCA (pANCA)
Churg–Strauss syndrome	**MPO-ANCA**
Coeliac disease	**Anti-endomysial** **Anti-tissue transglutaminase** **Anti-reticulin** **Anti-gliadin**

Diffuse cutaneous scleroderma	Rheumatoid factor Anti-nuclear **Anti-ScL-70** **Polymerase 1, 2 and 3**
Goodpasture's syndrome	**Anti-glomerular basement membrane**
Graves' disease	**Anti-TSH receptor** Anti-peroxidase
Hashimoto's thyroiditis	**TSH-receptor-blocking antibodies** Anti-peroxidase
Lambert–Eaton myasthenic syndrome	Anti-P/Q-type voltage-gated calcium channels
Limited cutaneous scleroderma	Rheumatoid factor Anti-nuclear **Anti-centromere**
Mixed connective tissue disease (overlap syndrome)	Anti-U1-RNP
Myasthenia gravis	Anti-nuclear **Anti-acetylcholine receptor antibodies**
Paraneoplastic conditions	Anti-YO Anti-Hu Anti-Ri Anti-MA Anti-CV2/CRMP5 Anti-amphiphysin
Pernicious anaemia	**Anti-parietal cell** **Anti-intrinsic factor**
Polyarteritis nodosa	**MPO-ANCA**

Polymyositis/dermatomyositis	Rheumatoid factor Anti-nuclear **Anti-Jo-1**
Primary biliary cirrhosis	**Anti-mitochondrial** (more particularly against pyruvate dehydrogenase complex type E2- and/or E3-binding protein)
Rheumatoid disease	**Rheumatoid factor** Anti-nuclear
Sjögren's syndrome	Rheumatoid factor Anti-nuclear **Anti-Ro (SS-A)** **Anti-La (SS-B)**
Systemic lupus erythematosus	**Double-stranded DNA** Rheumatoid factor Anti-nuclear Anti-Ro (SS-A) Anti-Sm Anti-U1-RNP Anti-cardiolipin
Wegener's syndrome	**Proteinase 3 anti-nuclear cytoplasmic antibody** (PR3-ANCA), also called cytoplasmic ANCA (cANCA)

IMAGING

9

With Dr Barry Kelly
Consultant Radiologist
Royal Victoria Hospital, Belfast
and Honorary Reader in Radiology,
The Queens University of Belfast

IMAGING

Interpretation of imaging investigations is such a vast topic that it forms a specialty within its own right. However, it is vital that students have a basic understanding of plain radiographs ('X-rays') and an appreciation of the more advanced imaging investigations used in modern medicine. Imaging plays a role in the everyday care of many patients and there is an expectation that junior doctors are competent in the assessment of commonly used films. Students should be well versed with chest and abdominal radiographs at the very least.

X-rays can feature in both written and clinical examinations and are suitable for use in most specialties.

This chapter does not aim to be a concise undergraduate textbook on radiology. Nor will it be an exhaustive description of characteristic radiological findings in common diseases or a gallery of images. It is a guide to approaching the interpretation of common X-rays. All X-rays included will serve to highlight clinical conditions in which radiology plays a pivotal role in diagnosis. The emphasis will be on 'ward films' – these are X-rays one might be expected to see or comment on during work on general medical and surgical wards. No film will be viewed in isolation without clinical information. As with all the data interpretation considered in this book, investigations should be assessed in the light of the clinical scenarios.

DON'T FORGET

Always interpret X-ray findings in a clinical context
Compare the images with old films if available

Interpreting the chest X-ray

The chest X-ray (CXR) is the single most requested imaging investigation and is also the most likely film to feature in an exam. It is the perfect prompt for questioning other aspects of a patient's condition and management. To be able to comment confidently on the film's findings, an appreciation of normality is required. Don't forget that a CXR is a two-dimensional representation of three-dimensional structures.

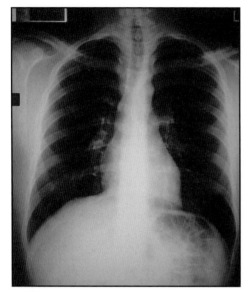

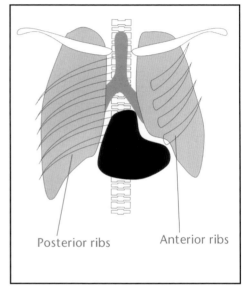

Posterior ribs   Anterior ribs

Fig 9.1   Fig 9.2

One may think of a CXR as a picture that contains five 'shades'. These shades represent five different 'tissues'.

The big two are:

1. Bone is WHITE

2. Gas is BLACK.

The others are:

3. Soft tissue is GREY

4. Fat is DARKER GREY.

And if anything man-made is on the film

5. It is BRIGHT WHITE.

Film specifics and technical factors

Before proceeding to interpret a CXR, always comment on film specifics and technical factors as shown in the boxes below.

FILM SPECIFICS (DETAILS)

Name of patient
Age and date of birth
Location of patient
Date taken
Film number (if applicable)

FILM TECHNICAL FACTORS

Type of projection (see box below)
Markings regarding any special techniques used (eg taken in expiration)
Rotation
Inspiration
Penetration

TYPES OF PROJECTION

Posteroanterior (PA): X-ray tube behind the patient and film against chest
Anteroposterior (AP): X-ray tube in front of the patient and film against back
Lateral: X-rays 'fired' through the patient from the side
Supine: the patient is lying on his or her back
Erect: the patient is upright
Semi-erect: the patient is upright but in an unideal position (usually an ill patient)
Mobile: the X-ray has been taken with a mobile x-ray unit (on the ward usually).

These descriptions can be combined. For example an acutely unwell patient who has a CXR taken on a ward may have a mobile, semi-erect AP film.

You might think of this part of the interpretation, like the safety announcement on an airplane, that one has heard many times: necessary to acknowledge, but tedious and of little consequence. However, this could not be further from the truth. Changes in these parameters can give the impression of abnormalities in the structures seen.

Assess the film in detail

Many students rush into interpretation and come out with statements such as: 'There it is – a big lump' or 'Oh I see the heart is big'. This approach will almost certainly lead to important details being missed. A structure is needed for thorough interpretation.

It is good practice to mention a clear-cut abnormality at the outset. A reasonable way to say this would be, 'The technical quality of the film is satisfactory. The most striking abnormality on initial assessment is …'.

The examiner will then expect the candidate to demonstrate an organised approach to looking at the rest of the film. Do not stop when one abnormality has been noted – there may be more to see ('the satisfaction of search').

DON'T FORGET
Don't stop looking

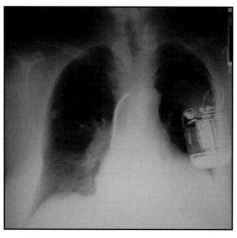

Fig 9.3

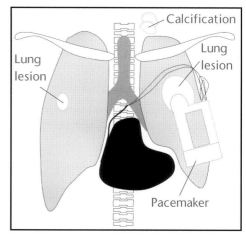

Fig 9.4

The structures below need to be considered in the interpretation of the film. As long as all review areas are covered one cannot be faulted over the order in which they are reviewed. It is fair to assume, however, that if one major abnormality is clearly seen from the beginning this structure or system should be commented on first.

Structures to assess on CXR

- Heart and major vessels
- Lungs and pleura
- Mediastinum (including hila)
- Bones and soft tissues.

Be particularly careful not to miss the following review areas. They should be specifically checked as abnormalities in these areas may be easily overlooked.

Review areas

- Costophrenic angles (1)
- Apices (2)
- Behind the heart (3)
- Below the diaphragms (4)
- Breast shadows (in females). (5)

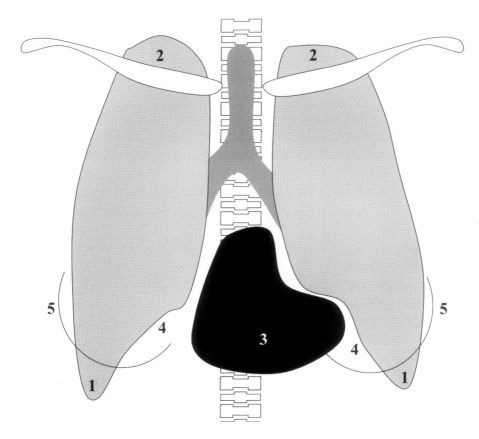

Fig 9.5: Schematic representation of structures seen on a CXR

Heart and major vessels

Assess:

- Size of heart
- Size of individual chambers of heart
- Size of pulmonary vessels
- Evidence of stents, clips, wires, valves, pacemakers
- Outline of aorta, inferior (IVC) and superior (SVC) vena cava.

DON'T FORGET

Do not comment on heart size on an AP chest X-ray

Lungs

Assess:

- Size
- Intrapulmonary pathology
- Vascular lung markings.

Pleura

Assess:

- Thickness or calcification
- Opposition against chest wall (ie is there a pneumothorax?).

Mediastinum (including hila)

Assess:

- Width of mediastinum
- Contour of mediastinum
- Size and density of hila
- Level and symmetry of hila.

Bones and soft tissues

Assess:

- Generalised bone disease, fractures and bony deposits
- Surgical emphysema
- Breast presence/absence and symmetry.

Abdominal X-ray

The abdominal X-ray (AXR) has more limited value in diagnosis than a CXR. This is partly the information that can realistically be extracted and the ready availability of more detailed cross sectional studies such as ultrasound and CT. The radiation exposure of an AXR compared with a CXR is also considerably higher. One AXR is equivalent to 35 CXRs.

The AXR is of most use in the patient with an acute abdomen. As with a CXR, such as an appreciation of normal structures is vital.

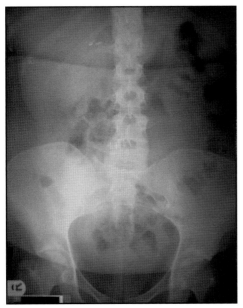

Fig 9.6

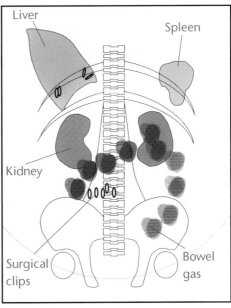

Fig 9.7

Film specifics and technical factors

The initial assessment of an AXR is similar to for a CXR.

FILM SPECIFICS	FILM TECHNICAL FACTORS
Name of patient	Type of projection (supine is standard)
Age and date of birth	Markings of any special techniques used
Location of patient	
Date taken	
Film number (if applicable)	

Assess the film in detail

A simple guide to interpretation is shown below. Working through these headings, one covers 'black bits', 'white bits', 'grey bits' and 'bright white bits' in turn.

'Black bits'
Intraluminal gas

Intraluminal gas can be normal. Extraluminal gas is abnormal. However, intraluminal gas can be abnormal if it is in the wrong place or if too much is seen.

The maximum normal diameter of the large bowel is 55 mm. Small bowel should be no more than 35 mm in diameter. The natural presence of gas within the bowel allows assessment of calibre – although the amount varies between individuals. The caecum is not considered to be dilated unless wider than 80 mm in diameter.

Large and small bowel may be distinguished by looking at bowel wall markings.

DON'T FORGET

The haustra of the large bowel extend only a third of the way across the diameter of the large bowel from each side.
The valvulae conniventes of the small bowel transverse the whole diameter

---

It is usual to see small volumes of gas throughout the gastrointestinal (GI) tract and the absence in one region may in itself represent pathology. For example, if gas is seen to the level of the splenic flexure and nothing is seen beyond this, a site of the obstruction at this site – a 'cut-off' point – is noted.

Extraluminal gas

When a bowel or any other gas-containing structure perforates, its contained gas becomes extraluminal. Extraluminal gas is never normal, but may be seen following intra-abdominal surgery, laparoscopy or endoscopic retrograde cholangiopancreatography (ERCP).

CAUSES OF EXTRALUMINAL GAS

Post abdominal surgery/ERCP
Perforation of viscus (eg bowel, stomach)
Abscess

DON'T FORGET

An erect CXR (not AXR) is the best projection to diagnose a pneumoperitoneum (gas in the peritoneal cavity)

'White bits'

Calcification

Calcified structures are often seen on an AXR. The main question is: 'Does their presence have any important implications?' Calcification can be broadly divided into three types:

1. Calcification that is an abnormal structure, eg gallstones, renal calculi, calcified splenic artery aneurysm.

2. Calcification that is within a normal structure, but represents pathology, eg nephrocalcinosis.

3. Calcification that is within a normal structure, but is not clinically significant, eg lymph node calcification.

Bones are normal 'white' structures. On the AXR they comprise mainly those of the thoracolumbar spine and pelvis. Findings can often be incidental.

'Grey bits'

Soft tissues

Soft tissues represent most of the contents of the abdomen and feature prominently in the AXR. However, these tissues are poorly seen when compared with other imaging techniques such as ultrasound, CT, or MRI.

The kidneys, spleen, liver and bladder (if filled) can be seen in addition to psoas muscle shadows and abdominal fat.

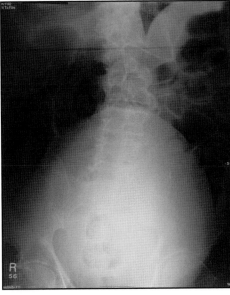

Fig 9.8

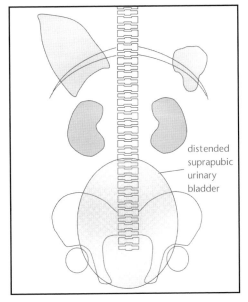

distended suprapubic urinary bladder

Fig 9.9

'Bright white bits'
Foreign bodies

Foreign bodies represent an interesting final observation. Objects that may be seen include ingested and rectal foreign bodies, as well as items in the path of the X-ray beam such as belt buckles, dress buttons and jewellery. Other objects may have been deliberately placed; for example, an aortic stent, an inferior vena cava filter or a suprapubic urinary catheter. Sterilisation clips and an intrauterine device are common findings in women.

Other imaging modalities

There is a range of other imaging modalities in regular use – the majority of which would not feature in undergraduate exams. Knowledge of their importance in diagnosis should be sufficient.

IONISING RADIATION TECHNIQUES	
Contrast studies (mostly barium)	Nuclear (radio nucleotide) imaging
Computed tomography (CT)	Fluoroscopy ('screening')

NON-IONISING RADIATION TECHNIQUES
Ultrasound
Magnetic resonance imaging (MRI)

Computed tomography (CT) imaging plays a diverse and pivotal role in contemporary clinical care.

This set of images of the same patient with an extensive bronchial carcinoma demonstrates the value of CT.

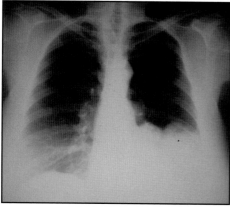

Fig 9.10

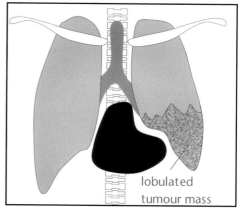

lobulated
tumour mass

Fig 9.11

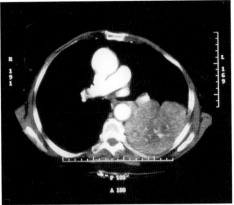

Fig 9.12

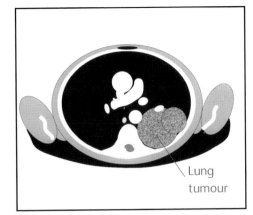

Fig 9.13

Case 62

This patient was admitted to the intensive care unit (ICU) following an accident. His CXR on day 5 of his stay is shown.

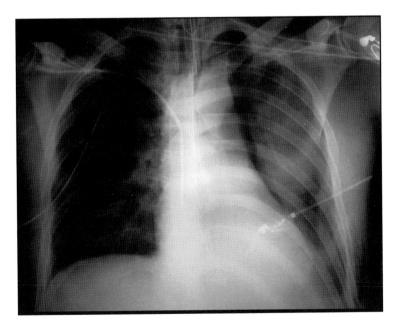

1. **Describe the different objects seen on the film.**

2. **What position should an endotracheal tube (ET) be in when correctly placed?**

Answer 62

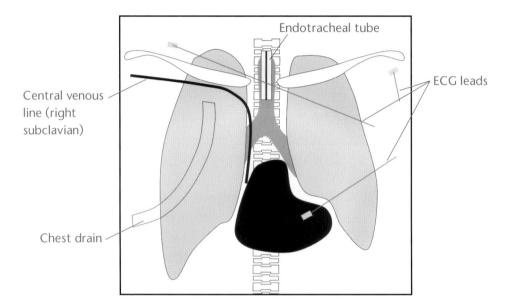

1. The following lines can be seen on the CXR (see line diagram)

   - endotracheal tube (ETT)

   - cardiac monitor leads

   - right subclavian central venous catheter ('line')

   - right apical chest drain.

   When assessing a chest x-ray, look for the presence and position of all lines before reviewing the rest of the film.

2. A correctly placed ETT should lie at least 2.5 cm above the carina. The ETT may slip into the right main bronchus during expiration if not positioned sufficiently above the carina.

Case 63

A 55-year-old man was admitted with acute abdominal pain and a CXR was performed.

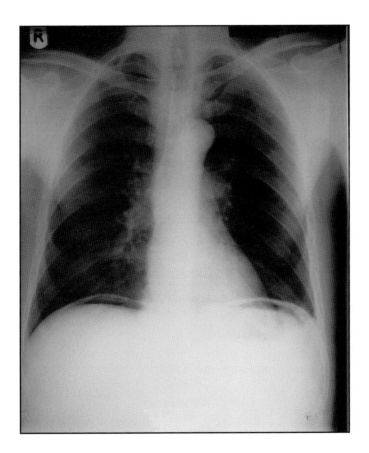

1. **What abnormality is seen on this film?**
2. **What projection has been used?**
3. **List some causes of this finding.**

Answer 63

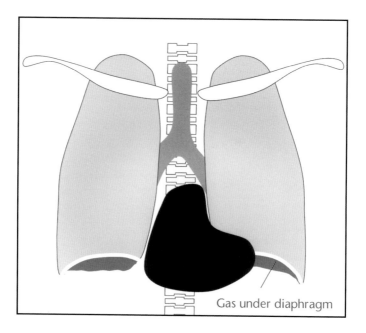

Gas under diaphragm

1. A radiolucent linear abnormality is noted inferior to the diaphragm bilaterally.

   Remember that gas on a plain X-ray is black so this must be gas in the abdomen.

   It is outside the bowel lumen – an abnormal finding. This is called a pneumoperitoneum.

2. This is an ERECT CXR. An erect film is invariably requested to assess for free gas within the abdomen (pneumoperitoneum).

3. The causes of pneumoperitoneum are listed on page 218 (see table 'causes of extraluminal gas').

Case 64

This 67-year-old man was admitted with shortness of breath and weight loss. A large lung mass was seen on his CXR. Other investigations confirmed that the lesion was a bronchial carcinoma in the left lower lobe of the lung.

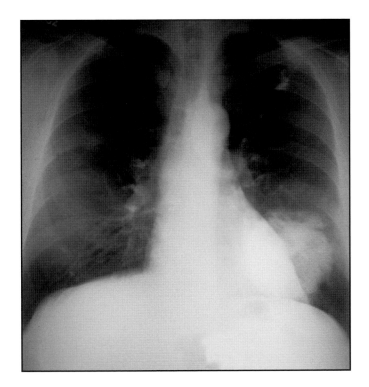

1. **What other findings might be seen on CXR in a patient with bronchial carcinoma?**

2. **What else could cause the appearance of a large mass like this on a CXR?**

3. **What other imaging investigation would be helpful?**

Answer 64

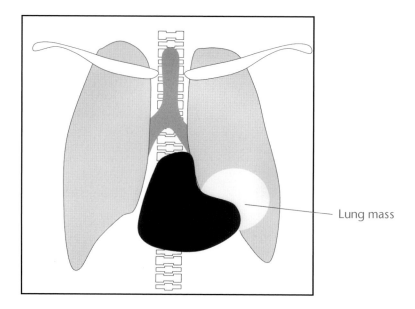

Lung mass

1. A large lung mass on a CXR in a smoker over 50 years of age should be regarded as a bronchial carcinoma until proven otherwise. Other features that may be seen on CXR with bronchial carcinoma include:

   - pleural effusion
   - lung collapse (due to endobronchial tumour)
   - pulmonary metastases
   - bony metastases (and pathological fracture)
   - secondary pneumonia
   - lymphangitis carcinomatosis
   - enlarged lymph nodes (hilar and paratracheal).

2. Causes of a lung mass on CXR include:

   - bronchial carcinoma
   - pulmonary metastasis
   - round pneumonia
   - lung hamartoma

- encysted pleural effusion

- rheumatoid nodule

- lung abscess (usually cavitating).

3. Computed tomography of the chest would image the mass in greater detail. It will also help in the assessment of lymphadenopathy and provide evidence of local or metastatic spread.

See below an example of a chest CT in a patient with a lung mass (a different patient to that shown in the CXR above). Greater detail of the mass and its relation to other structures can be observed.

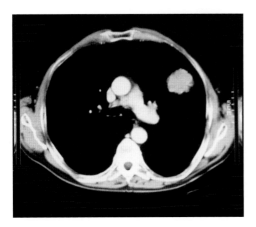 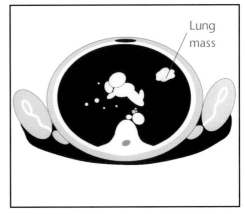

Lung mass

Case 65

This 34-year-old man is admitted with shortness of breath and fever.

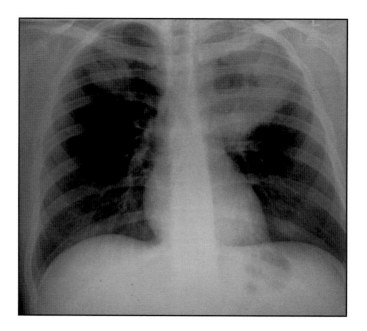

1. **Describe the findings on this CXR.**

2. **What are the potential causes of such an appearance?**

Answer 65

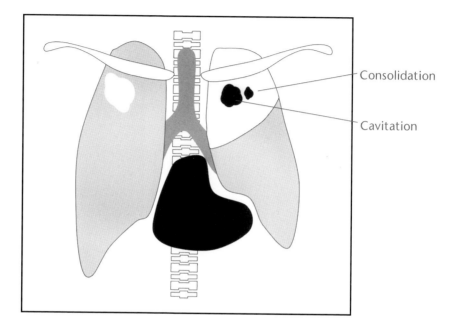

Consolidation

Cavitation

1. There is a large cavitating lesion in the upper lobe of the left lung.
   Increased shadowing is seen in the upper lobe with a central area of
   radiolucency. The radiolucent area represents gas within an area of
   consolidation within the lung. In the right lung there is a similar smaller
   lesion in the upper lobe.

2. The differential diagnosis for a cavitating lung lesion is:
   - bronchial carcinoma (especially squamous cell carcinoma)
   - pulmonary metastasis
   - tuberculosis
   - cavitating pneumonia
   - lung abscess
   - vasculitic disease (eg Wegener's granulomatosis)
   - lung infarction
   - rheumatoid nodule.

Case 66

A 32-year-old man attends A&E complaining of shortness of breath and the development of a rash on her shins.

A CXR was requested.

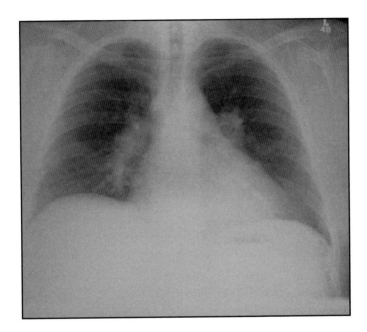

1. **Outline any abnormal findings seen on this film.**

2. **Give a differential diagnosis for this appearance.**

Answer 66

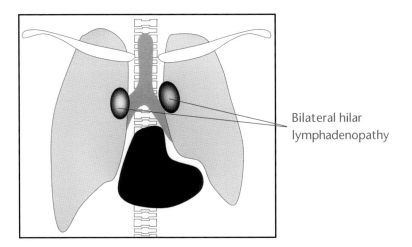

Bilateral hilar
lymphadenopathy

1. The mediastinal contour is abnormal. There is bilateral hilar enlargement.
   When bilateral hilar enlargement is observed the three important potential
   diagnoses are sarcoidosis, lymphoma (enlarged nodes) and pulmonary
   hypertension (enlarged pulmonary vessels). You should therefore pay special
   attention to the lungs to assess for the presence of other signs that might
   point to one of these diagnoses.

DISEASE	SUPPORTING FEATURES
Sarcoidosis	Interstitial fibrotic change
Lymphoma	Enlargement of other nodes (para-tracheal)
Pulmonary hypertension	Peripheral pruning Chronic lung disease (cause of secondary pulmonary hypertension)

2. Causes of bilateral hilar enlargement include:

   - sarcoidosis
   - lymphoma
   - pulmonary hypertension (primary and secondary)
   - metastatic nodal disease.

Case 67

This 55-year-old man attended his local hospital feeling increasingly short of breath over the past week. He has lost 1 stone in weight recently. He is a smoker of 60 pack-years. His CXR is shown.

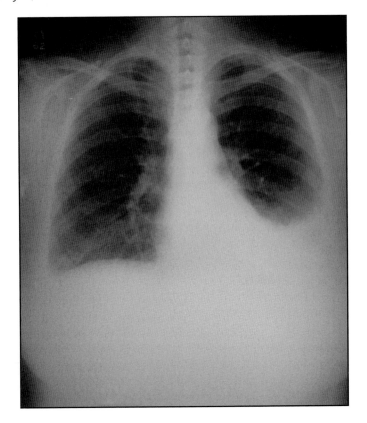

1. **Describe the appearances on the CXR.**

2. **List the causes of this finding, and state the most likely cause in this patient.**

3. **What other simple test may assist in forming a diagnosis?**

Answer 67

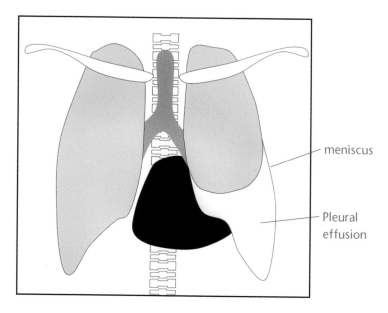

1. There is an area of increased radio-opacity at the lower left hemithorax. The edge can be seen to taper at the lateral aspect of the chest, forming a meniscus. There is no shift of mediastinal structures. This is a moderately sized left-sided pleural effusion.

2. Unilateral pleural effusions, and causes are mostly exudates. These include:

    - malignant tumours (both primary and metastatic disease)
    - parapneumonic
    - pulmonary embolus or infarction
    - rheumatoid disease.

   A malignant effusion would be most likely in this patient because of his weight loss and smoking history.

3. A diagnostic pleural aspiration could be performed. This will help distinguish whether the effusion is an exudate or transudate based on the protein content (see page 159 for details).

   In this case, malignant cells may be identified when the pleural fluid is examined cytologically.

Case 68

This 69-year-old woman was admitted to the surgical ward with malodorous vomiting and a distended abdomen.

An AXR was taken while she was in A&E.

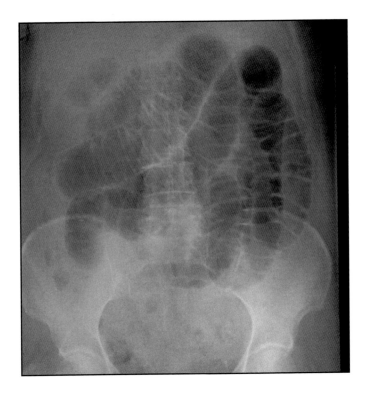

1. **Describe the findings on the AXR.**

2. **What are the causes of this abnormality?**

Answer 68

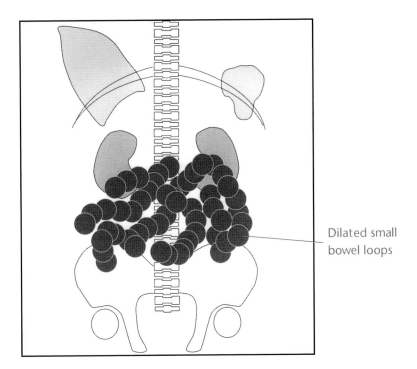

Dilated small
bowel loops

1. Multiple dilated small bowel loops. The bowel measures 4 cm in diameter
   and is located in the centre of the film. Multiple loops suggest that the
   obstruction lies within the lower small bowel. These findings are in keeping
   with a diagnosis of small bowel obstruction.

FEATURES OF SMALL BOWEL OBSTRUCTION

Bowel lies in centre of the film
Markings seen across the bowel wall (valvulae conniventes)
Several loops (more loops the lower the obstruction)

2. Causes of small bowel obstruction include (commonest first):

   - adhesions

   - hernia

   - intraluminal cause (obstructing mass).

Case 69

This 55-year-old man has been attending hospital for several years with various problems. He is admitted on this occasion with abdominal pain.

An AXR was performed.

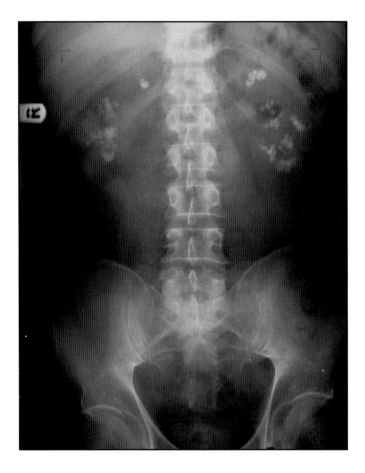

Describe the film and give a diagnosis.

Answer 69

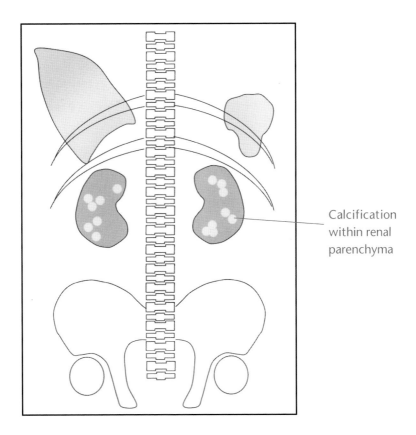

Calcification
within renal
parenchyma

Diffuse calcification is seen projecting over the renal outlines bilaterally. The calcification appears to be within the parenchyma of the kidneys. These findings are in keeping with nephrocalcinosis.

Case 70

This 46-year-old retired firefighter has become increasingly short of breath over the past 6 months. He complains of a dry cough. Pulmonary function tests and CXR were requested.

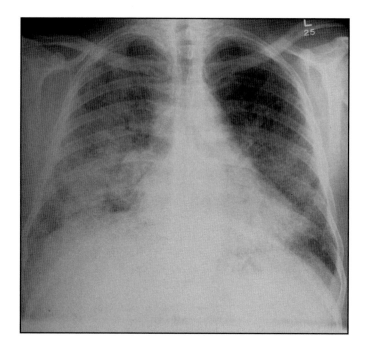

1.   **How would you describe the lungs on this CXR?**

2.   **What are the possible causes for these findings?**

3.   **What are his pulmonary function tests likely to demonstrate?**

Answer 70

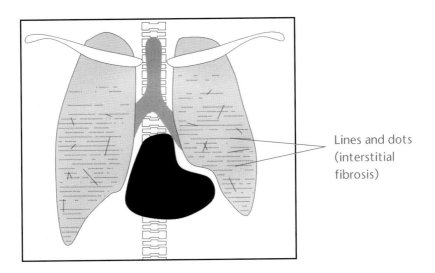

Lines and dots
(interstitial
fibrosis)

1. Diffuse reticulonodular ('lines and dots') shadowing is seen in both lungs. This has lower zone predominance.

2. The appearances of this CXR are of pulmonary (interstitial) fibrosis.

   The causes may be divided according to whether the fibrosis predominantly affects the upper or lower zones.

MEMORY AID	
Upper lobe fibrosis **(mnemonic = BREAST)** **B**erylliosis (uncommon) **R**adiation fibrosis **E**xtrinsic allergic alveolitis **A**nkylosing spondylitis **S**arcoidosis **T**uberculosis	**Lower lobe fibrosis** Cryptogenic fibrosing alveolitis Drug induced (eg amiodarone, methotrexate) Asbestosis Connective tissue diseases (eg rheumatoid diseases)

3. Spirometry would demonstrate a restrictive pattern (see page 326 for further details).

Case 71

This 47-year-old man attends outpatient clinic with the complaint of retro-sternal chest pain. He has attended his GP several times over the past month with this recurring complaint.

The SHO at the clinic requests a CXR.

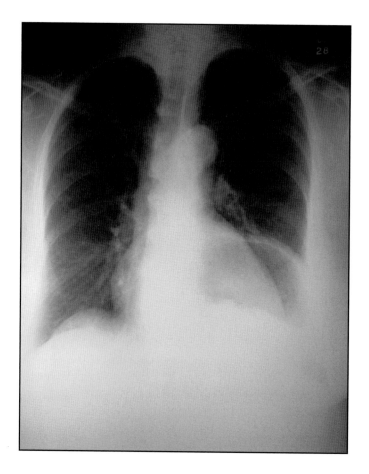

1. **Write a short report of your findings.**
2. **What else could give this appearance on a CXR?**

Answer 71

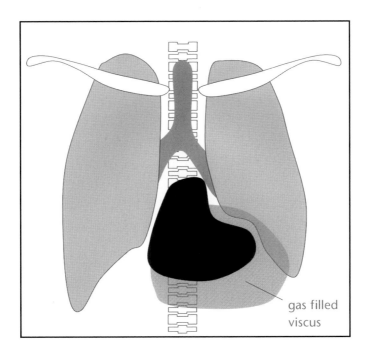

gas filled
viscus

1. A large retrocardiac gas filled viscus is seen. A gas–fluid interface is noted. These findings most likely represent a large hiatus hernia.

2. Other causes that could potentially give a similar appearance are:

    - a dilated oesophagus (eg achalasia)
    - surgically transposed stomach in the thorax (after oesophageal surgery)
    - herniated bowel in the thorax
    - an abscess cavity.

Case 72

This 72-year-old man was admitted to hospital with shortness of breath while on holiday in the Lake District. He has a past history of a myocardial infarction (MI) 7 years previously.

A CXR was requested by a nurse practitioner in A&E. No previous X-rays are available for comparison.

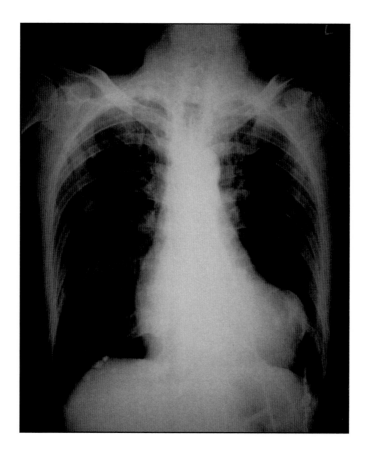

1. **Describe this CXR, as if you were on the telephone to your senior colleague.**

2. **What other findings might be noted on a CXR after an MI?**

Answer 72

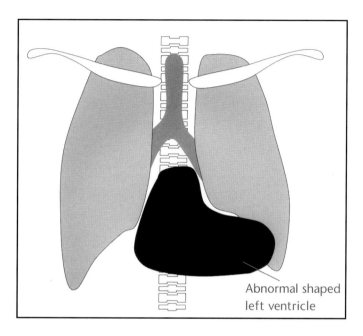

Abnormal shaped
left ventricle

1. The heart is enlarged. The left ventricle is abnormal in size and shape. Curvilinear calcification is seen within the wall of the left ventricle. The appearances are in keeping with a ventricular aneurysm.

2. Potential findings on CXR following MI include:

   - acute pulmonary oedema
   - cardiomegaly
   - pericardial effusion
   - iatrogenic objects (sternotomy wires, surgical clips)
   - ventricular aneurysm (late).

CARDIOLOGY

10

CARDIOLOGY

Electrocardiography

The electrocardiogram (ECG) is one of the most important commonly requested tests in medical practice.

> **DON'T FORGET**
>
> If possible, always compare ECGs with previous tracings

Components of an ECG tracing

A standard ECG comprises 12 individual tracings (called leads). An ECG machine produces these tracings by comparing electrical signals from ten sensors. Six are placed on the chest and one on each of the four limbs. By convention, the tracings are given standard names, and each tracing represents an electrical signal from a particular part of the heart. V1, V2, V3, V4, V5 and V6 'look at' the heart in a horizontal plane. Each of these tracings represents the electrical signal detected at one of the chest sensors; aVL, aVF, aVR, I, II and III look at the heart in a vertical plane.

LEAD	LOOKS AT
V1, V2, V3 and V4	Anterior surface (right ventricle and septum)
V5, V6, aVL and I	Lateral surface (left ventricle)
II, III and aVF	Inferior surface
aVR	Right atrium

In a patient having an acute myocardial infarction, it is therefore possible to determine which part of the heart is affected by looking at which leads show changes.

If any individual lead is looked at in detail, various peaks and troughs will be noted. These represent electrical activity at various times in the cardiac cycle. It is sometimes difficult to see every detail on each tracing. Names are attached to particular parts of the tracing as follows.

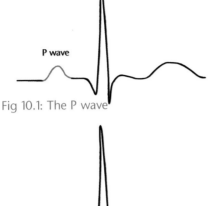

P wave

Fig 10.1: The P wave

The first bump in a tracing is called a 'P wave'. This represents the electrical activity associated with depolarisation of the atria. There is a further electrical signal associated with atrial repolarisation, but this cannot usually be seen on an ECG, since the small electrical signal is overshadowed by the much more powerful ventricular activity.

Q wave

Fig 10.2: The Q wave

Following along from the P wave, a downward dip in the tracing is known as a Q wave. This may or may not be present.

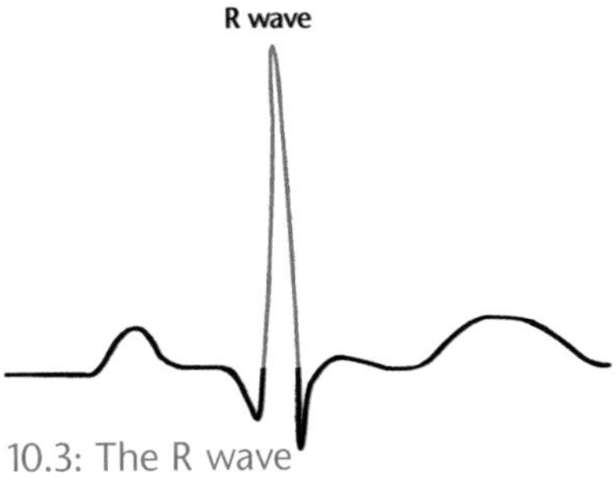

R wave

Fig 10.3: The R wave

The first upward peak after the P wave is known as an R wave.

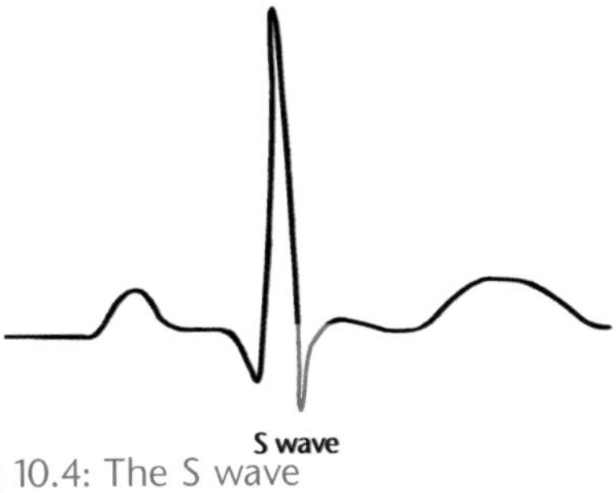

Any dip below the baseline following an R wave is called an S wave.

S wave

Fig 10.4: The S wave

The Q, R and S waves are known collectively as the QRS complex. This represents ventricular depolarisation.

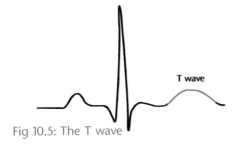

T wave

Fig 10.5: The T wave

Following the QRS complex, an upward deflection in the tracing is known as a T wave. This represents ventricular repolarisation. T waves are followed by P waves, and the cycle is complete.

Interpreting an ECG

The following aspects should be addressed when interpreting an ECG.

Heart rate	QRS complexes
Heart rhythm	ST segment
Cardiac axis	Q–T interval
P waves	T waves

Heart rate

ECGs are printed on squared paper. This paper usually runs through the ECG machine at a standard rate (25 mm/s). If, for some reason, the machine is set to run at a different speed, interpretation is more difficult.

DON'T FORGET

Always check that the paper speed is at 25 mm per second

At this speed, on a horizontal axis, each small square represents 0.04 second, and each large square (which is five small squares wide) represents 0.2 second.

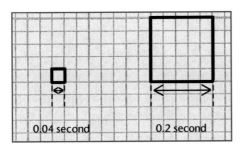

Fig 10.6: Standard squared paper used when recording ECGs

The ventricular rate is calculated by looking at the distance between consecutive QRS complexes. Usually the distance between R waves is analysed.

When there are a number of large squares between each R wave, the ventricular rate is most easily calculated by counting the number of large squares between each R wave and dividing this number into 300.

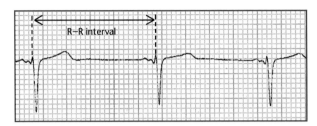

Fig 10.7: Measuring the R–R interval

In the ECG shown, there are approximately five large squares between each R wave. The ventricular rate is therefore 300 ÷ 5 = 60 beats per minute.

When the ventricular rhythm is more rapid, counting large squares can prove difficult. In such instances, the number of small squares between consecutive R waves is counted, and this number divided into 1500.

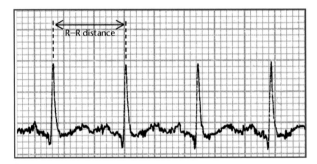

Fig 10.8: Measuring the R–R interval with a faster heart rate

In the example, there are 12 small squares between each R wave. The ventricular rate is therefore 1500 ÷ 12 = 125 beats per minute.

Ventricular rate (beats per minute) = 300 ÷ number of large squares between R waves

OR

Ventricular rate (beats per minute) = 1500 ÷ number of small squares between R waves

A heart rate of less than 60 beats per minute is termed bradycardia. A rate of greater than 100 beats per minute is tachycardia.

If the heart rhythm is irregular, calculate the rate using the number of squares between several R waves. Divide the answer to obtain an average R–R interval.

Heart rhythm

There are several heart rhythms that you will be expected to recognise. To assess rhythm, look for P waves and their relationship to QRS complexes. Remember that normally one P wave should be followed by one QRS complex.

Sinus rhythm

Sinus rhythm describes a normal heart rhythm in which electrical signals begin in the sinus node. A P wave should precede each QRS complex, and be at a normal, fixed interval from it. The P–R interval is used to measure the interval between P waves and QRS complexes. It is measured by counting the number of squares between the start of the P wave and the start of the QRS complex. This distance should be between three and five small squares.

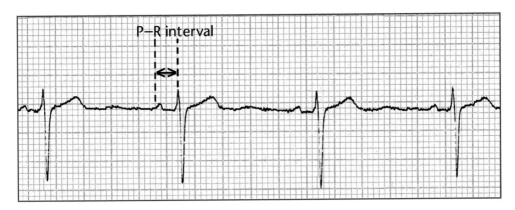

Fig 10.9: Normal sinus rhythm illustrating the P–R interval

- Sinus tachycardia describes sinus rhythm at a rate of over 100 beats per minute.

- Sinus bradycardia describes sinus rhythm at less than 60 beats per minute.

- Sinus arrhythmia is the term used to describe the normal variation in heart rate with respiration. Normally, the heart rate increases on inspiration.

In sinus arrhythmia, the heart rate **IN**creases on **IN**spiration

Atrial fibrillation

This is the term used to describe erratic electrical activity in the atria. In this condition, no P waves are seen, and the ECG baseline commonly shows irregularity. QRS complexes occur irregularly.

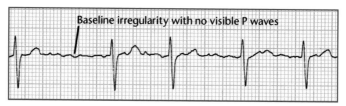

Fig 10.10: Atrial fibrillation

Atrial flutter

This condition is similar to atrial fibrillation in many ways. However, the ECG shows the presence of F waves (flutter waves). The baseline of the ECG therefore adopts a 'saw-toothed' appearance. Atrial flutter may occur with a fixed degree of atrioventricular block, for example three-to-one block. This means that, for every three flutter waves, there would be one QRS complex. Alternatively, the rhythm may have variable block, where the number of flutter waves preceding each QRS complex varies from beat to beat.

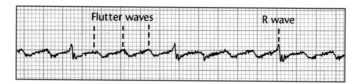

Fig 10.11: Atrial flutter

Heart block

Heart block describes a problem with conduction between the atria and ventricles. There are various types.

First-degree heart block

A P wave precedes each QRS complex, but the P–R interval is prolonged (more than five small squares). The P–R interval remains constant from beat to beat.

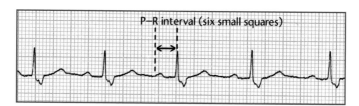

Fig 10.12: First-degree heart block

Second-degree heart block

There are three main types:

1. Mobitz type I (Wenckebach phenomenon)
   This rhythm runs in cycles, and will be identified if the P–R interval is studied. The first P–R interval in a cycle is often normal. With each successive heart beat, the P–R interval lengthens. Eventually, there will be a P wave with no following QRS complex. The cycle then begins again.

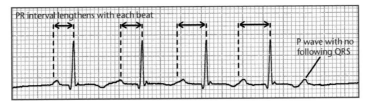

Fig 10.13: Mobitz type I heart block

2. Mobitz type II
   In this rhythm, the P–R interval is constant. Its duration may be normal or prolonged. However, periodically there will be no conduction between the atria and ventricles, and there will be a P wave with no associated QRS complex.

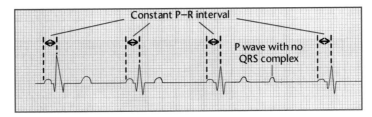

Fig 10.14: Mobitz type II heart block

3. Fixed degrees of atrioventricular block
   These rhythms are described as two-to-one, three-to-one, four-to-one block, etc. In two-to-one block, two P waves are found for every QRS complex. The QRS complexes are wide with these rhythms (see below for more details).

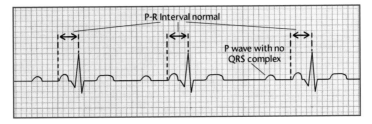

Fig 10.15: Two-to-one atrioventricular block

Third-degree heart block

In this condition, there is no functioning electrical connection between the atria and ventricles. P waves and QRS complexes will be seen, but these will have no constant relationship to each other. If you suspect this rhythm, take a sheet of paper and lay it alongside the ECG in question. Mark on the paper the position of the P waves. Next, move your paper so that the first mark you have made lines up with the first QRS complex. You will see that the P waves and QRS complexes are completely dissociated. The QRS complex arises because of intrinsic pacemaker activity below the atrioventricular node.

Note that QRS complexes can be normal in width or wide (see below).

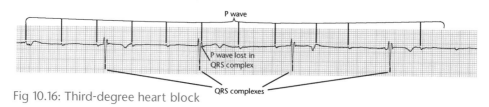

Fig 10.16: Third-degree heart block

Cardiac axis

This is an arbitrary concept used to describe the average direction of electrical activity in the heart. Normally, electrical energy moves from the upper right heart border towards the apex. In various disease states, the cardiac axis can shift.

The cardiac axis can be assessed by looking at leads I, II and III, and determining whether they are predominantly upgoing or downgoing.

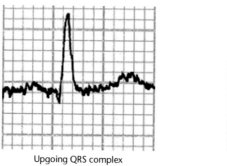

Upgoing QRS complex

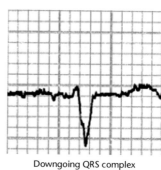

Downgoing QRS complex

Fig 10.17: Upgoing and downgoing QRS complexes

AXIS	LEAD I	LEAD II	LEAD III
Normal	Upgoing	Upgoing	Upgoing (or downgoing)
Right axis deviation	Downgoing	Upgoing	Upgoing
Left axis deviation	Upgoing	Downgoing	Downgoing

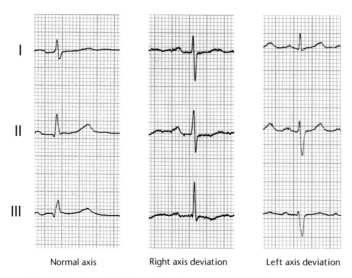

Normal axis   Right axis deviation   Left axis deviation

Fig 10.18: Leads I, II and III showing a normal axis, right axis deviation and left axis deviation

P waves

Look at leads II and V1 for the best views of P waves. Assess their size and shape. P waves should not exceed the maximum dimensions shown in the diagram. Always make sure that an ECG has been correctly calibrated before commenting on the heights of peaks. The standard calibration is 10 mm = 1 mV.

DON'T FORGET

Always check that an ECG is calibrated to 10 mm = 1 mV

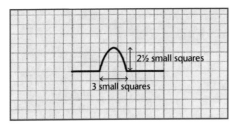

Fig 10.19: Normal P-wave dimensions

- P pulmonale describes tall, peaked P waves. These occur in conditions when the right atrium becomes enlarged.
- P mitrale describes wide P waves that are often bifid. This may be seen with mitral stenosis.

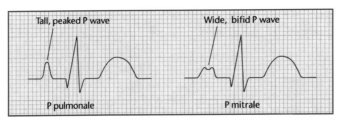

Fig 10.20: P pulmonale and P mitrale

MEMORY AID

In P **P**ulmonale, the P waves are **P**eaked
In P **M**itrale, the P waves are bifid and look like the letter **M**

QRS complexes
Q waves
Look at the location and size of Q waves. The maximum dimensions of Q waves should not exceed those shown in the diagram.

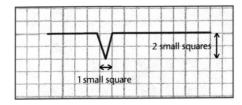

Fig 10.21: Q-wave maximum dimensions

Because of the direction taken by electrical signals in the heart, small Q waves may normally be seen in leads looking at the lateral aspect of the heart (V5, V6, aVL and I). Large Q waves or Q waves in other locations are abnormal, and indicate the presence of scar tissue in the heart (for example, following a myocardial infarction).

Height of R and S waves

Much information can be gleaned by looking at the height of R and S waves. The most common abnormality detected is left ventricular hypertrophy. If the sum of the height of the S wave in V1 (in mm) and the height of the R wave in V6 (in mm) is greater than 35 mm, it is probable that left ventricular hypertrophy is present.

There are several causes of very small complexes, the most common being pericardial effusions, pericarditis and emphysematous lungs.

QRS duration

A normal QRS complex should be less than three small squares wide.

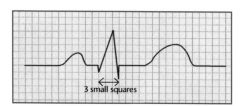

3 small squares

Fig 10.22: Normal maximum QRS complex duration

Wide complexes indicate abnormal conduction through the ventricles. Normally, electrical signals are carried through the ventricular muscle in specialised conducting tissue – the bundle of His and its left and right branches. Problems in this conducting tissue result in electrical impulses being carried more slowly through non-specialised cardiac tissue. This results in widening of the QRS complex. You should be able to recognise the typical ECG features of both problems in both the left and right bundle branches (left and right bundle branch-block).

In right bundle-branch block (RBBB), two upward deflections (ie two R waves) are seen in the QRS complex in V1. This is known as an RSR pattern. A deep S wave is seen in V6.

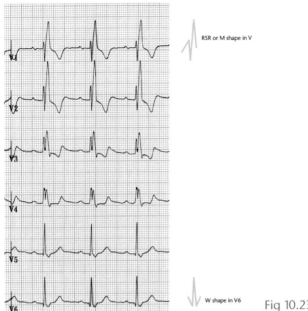

RSR or M shape in V

W shape in V6

Fig 10.23: Right bundle-branch block

In left bundle-branch block (LBBB), an RSR pattern may be seen in V6. New LBBB may be a sign of a myocardial infarction. When LBBB is present the only other information that can be obtained from the ECG is the ventricular rate and heart rhythm.

Do not attempt to comment on the ST segment when LBBB is present

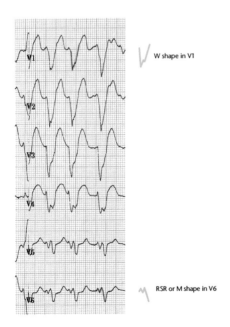

W shape in V1

RSR or M shape in V6

Fig 10.24: Left bundle-branch block

Remember the name William Morrow, to remind you that:
In LBBB, there is a W shape to the QRS complex in V1 and an M shape
to the complex in V6
In RBBB, there is an M shape to the QRS complex in V1 and a W shape
to the complex in V6

	V1						**V6**
LBBB	**W**	I	**L**	**L**	I	A	**M**
RBBB	**M**	O	**R**	**R**		O	**W**

ST segment

The ST segment is that part of a tracing that lies between the QRS complex
and the T wave.

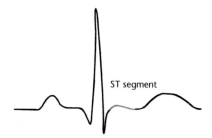

ST segment

Fig 10.25: The ST segment

Normally, the ST segment should be horizontal and isoelectric (ie lying on the
baseline of the tracing).

The ST segment may be elevated. The commonest causes for this are
myocardial infarction (where ST elevation occurs in the heart leads 'looking at'
damaged parts of the heart) and pericarditis (where ST elevation occurs in
most or all ECG leads). The ST elevation associated with myocardial infarction
is typically convex upwards, and in worst-case scenarios can look like a
tombstone. ST elevation is concave (saddle-shaped) in pericarditis.

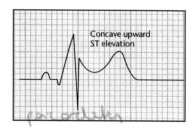
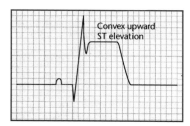

Fig 10.26: Convex and concave ST elevation

ST elevation that persists over weeks and months after a myocardial infarction commonly signifies the presence of a ventricular aneurysm.

Horizontal ST depression may represent cardiac ischaemia, and may be seen during episodes of angina pectoris. ST depression may also be the only sign of a non-ST elevation myocardial infarction (NSTEMI).

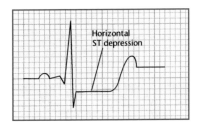

Fig 10.27: Horizontal ST depression

When ST depression in lateral chest leads is seen alongside features in keeping with left ventricular hypertrophy, this is called a strain pattern, and is a feature of hypertensive cardiac damage. It can be difficult to differentiate from changes associated with ischaemia.

Down-sloping ST depression (often called 'reverse tick' ST depression) is seen in patients on digoxin.

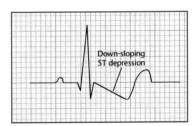

Fig 10.28: Down-sloping ST depression

Q–T interval

The Q–T interval is the distance from the start of the QRS complex to the end of the T wave. Long Q–T intervals predispose to cardiac dysrhythmias. The Q–T interval varies with heart rate, but should in general not be more than 2 large squares in duration.

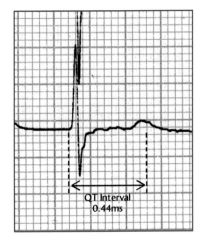

Fig 10.29: Prolonged Q–T interval

To make matters a little more complicated, the Q–T interval increases as the heart rate decreases. Thus bradycardia can be associated with an apparently long Q–T interval. To correct for this, Bazett's correction is applied to the Q–T interval to take the heart rate into account. The corrected Q–T interval (Q–Tc) is calculated as follows:

$$Q\text{–}Tc = \frac{Q\text{–}T}{\sqrt{R\text{–}R}}$$

where R–R is the number of seconds between consecutive R waves.

This value should generally be less than 0.45 second.

T wave

The final stage in ECG interpretation should be to look at the T waves. T waves may be upright or inverted (upside down). They are generally less than two-thirds of the height of their neighbouring R wave, and should not be more than two large squares tall.

Inverted T waves are normally seen in leads aVR and III. They may also be seen in lead V1 ± V2, but not V2 alone. T-wave inversion in other leads may be of little consequence, but is often a sign of cardiac ischaemia, or of NSTEMI.

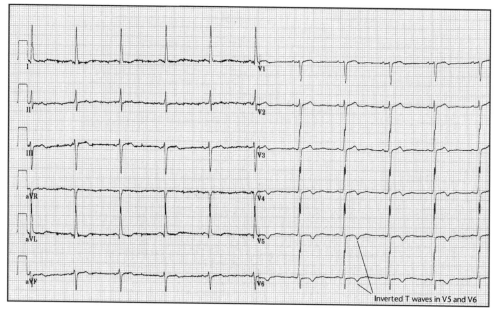

Inverted T waves in V5 and V6

Fig 10.30: 12-lead ECG with T-wave inversion in the lateral chest leads

T–wave changes often accompany changes in the serum potassium level. Typical findings are shown in the table.

HYPERKALAEMIA	HYPOKALAEMIA
Tall, tented T waves	Flat, broad T waves
Loss of P waves	ST depression
QRS complex broadening	Long Q–T interval
Sine-wave-shaped ECG	Ventricular dysrhythmias
Cardiac arrest rhythms	

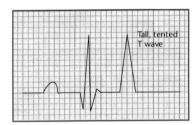

Fig 10.31: T waves in hyperkalaemia

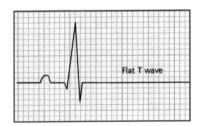

Fig 10.32: T waves in hypokalaemia

Summary

When interpreting an ECG, always use the following headings:

Heart rate	QRS complexes
Heart rhythm	ST segment
Cardiac axis	Q–T interval
P waves	T waves

Case 73

A 50-year-old manager presents to the accident and emergency department complaining of chest pain. He is very worried that he may be having a heart attack, since his brother had one last year. He has no other risk factors for cardiac disease. On further questioning, he describes doing heavy work in his garden on the previous day. Examination reveals an anxious man with tenderness on either side of the sternum. An ECG is performed.

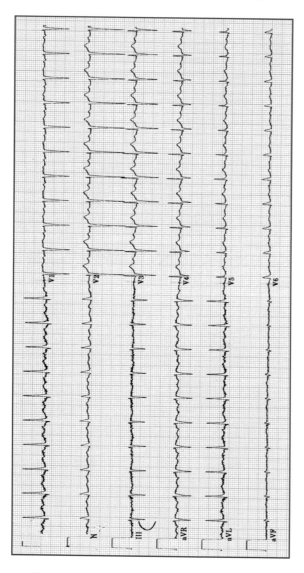

What is your interpretation?

Answer 73

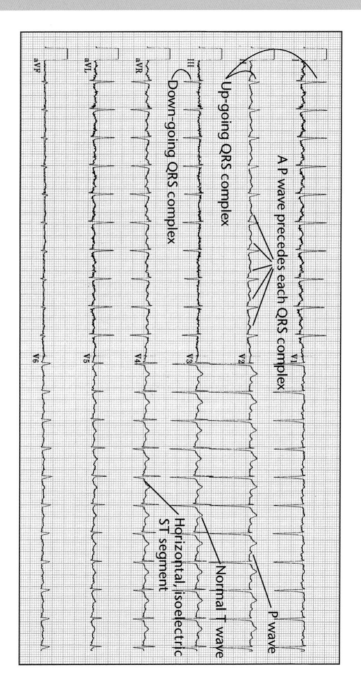

A P wave precedes each QRS complex

Up-going QRS complex

Down-going QRS complex

P wave

Normal T wave

Horizontal, isoelectric ST segment

V1
V2
V3
V4
V5
V6
aVR
aVL
aVF
III

Heart rate

There are 12 small squares between consecutive R waves. The ventricular rate is therefore 1500 ÷ 12 = 125 beats per minute.

Heart rhythm

A P wave precedes each QRS complex. The P–R interval is normal (four small squares) and does not vary from beat to beat. The rhythm is sinus rhythm.

Cardiac axis

Leads I and II are upgoing. Lead III is downgoing. The axis is normal.

P waves

P waves are of normal size and shape.

QRS complexes

There are no abnormal Q waves. The R and S waves are of normal height. The QRS complex is of normal duration (two small squares).

ST segment

The ST segment is horizontal and isoelectric.

Q–T interval

The Q–T interval is normal (1.5 large squares).

T waves

T waves are normal in size and shape.

Conclusion – sinus tachycardia. The most likely cause of this is anxiety. Sinus tachycardia is the commonest ECG finding in patients with a pulmonary embolism, so this diagnosis should be considered. However, in this case, history and examination point to the true cause of this man's chest pain – muscular strain.

Case 74

A 70-year-old woman with a history of a myocardial infarction presents with palpitations that are of recent onset. Her ECG is shown.

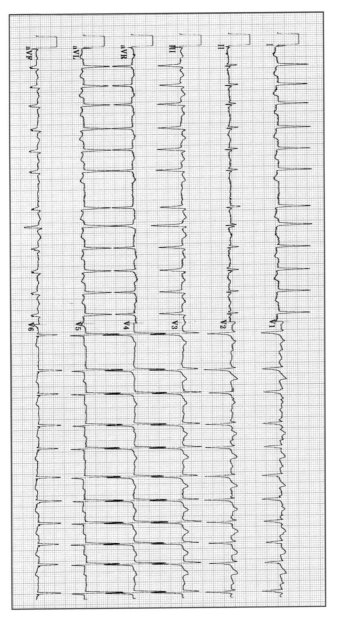

How would you interpret it?

Answer 74

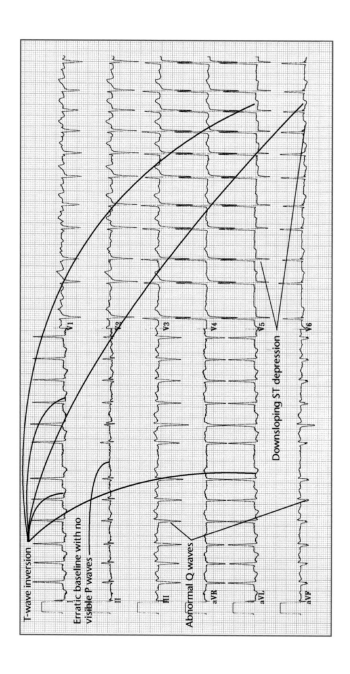

Heart rate

There are nine small squares between the first two consecutive R waves in lead I. The ventricular rate is therefore 1500 ÷ 9 = 167 beats per minute. However, since the rhythm is clearly irregular, a more accurate assessment of heart rate can be made by measuring the distance between the first and eleventh R waves and dividing this distance by 10 to find the average R–R interval.

By this method, there are approximately 20.5 large squares between the first and eleventh R waves. The average R–R interval is therefore 2.05 large squares. The heart rate is 300 ÷ 2.05 = 146 beats per minute.

Heart rhythm

No P waves are visible. The baseline is erratic. QRS complexes occur irregularly. The rhythm is atrial fibrillation.

Cardiac axis

Leads I and II are upgoing. Lead III is downgoing. The axis is normal.

P waves

No P waves are visible.

QRS complexes

There are abnormal Q waves in leads III and aVF, indicating a previous inferior myocardial infarction. The R and S waves are of normal height. The QRS complex is of normal duration (two small squares).

ST segment

The ST segment is horizontal and isoelectric in leads II, III, aVR, aVF, V1, V2 and V3. There is slight downsloping ST depression in the other leads, most marked in I and V6.

Q–T interval

The Q–T interval is normal (seven small squares).

T waves

T waves are normal in size. There is T-wave inversion in leads I, aVL, V5 and V6.

Conclusion – atrial fibrillation with a ventricular rate of 146 beats per minute. Inferior Q waves. There is downsloping ST elevation and T-wave inversion in the leads looking at the lateral aspect of the heart. The patient may be on digoxin, but the T-wave changes probably indicate ischaemia. This may be related to the rapid heart rate, and may disappear if the rate is slowed. This woman's palpitations are due to a sudden onset of atrial fibrillation.

Case 75

A 74-year-old man is admitted complaining of dizziness. He has had several myocardial infarctions in the past. Clinical examination reveals a pulse rate of 30 beats per minute, and a blood pressure of 62/46 mmHg. An ECG is performed.

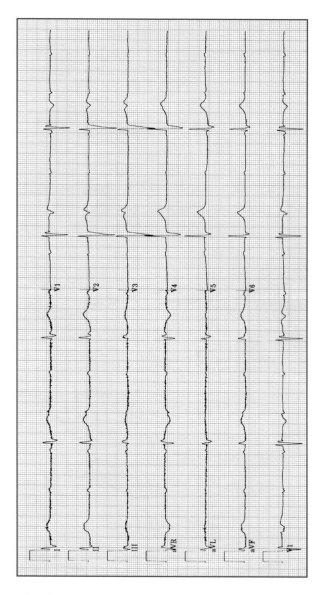

What does it show?

Answer 75

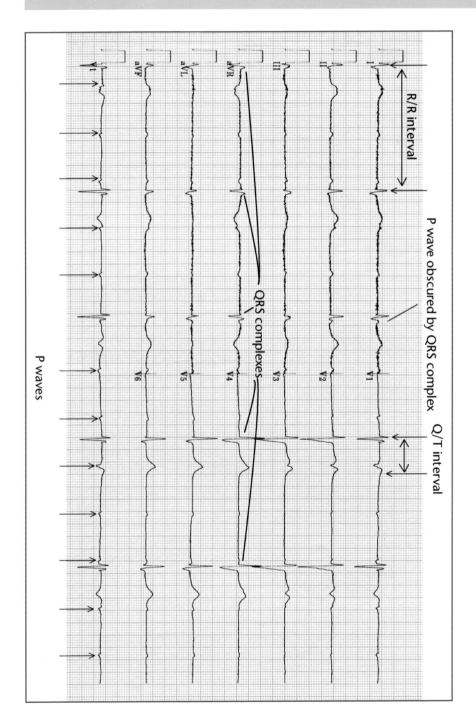

Heart rate

There are 10 big squares between consecutive R waves. The ventricular rate is therefore 300 ÷ 10 = 30 beats per minute.

Heart rhythm

P waves are seen, but these show no consistent relationship with the QRS complexes. The P waves and QRS complexes are completely dissociated. The rhythm is third-degree heart block.

Cardiac axis

Leads I, II and III are all upgoing. The axis is normal.

P waves

P waves are of normal size and shape. One P wave is difficult to see because it is obscured by a simultaneous QRS complex.

QRS complexes

There are no abnormal Q waves. The QRS complexes are narrow (two small squares). This indicates that the electrical signal to the ventricles is originating in specialised conducting tissue. The R and S waves are of normal height.

ST segment

The ST segment is horizontal and isoelectric.

QT interval

The QT interval is prolonged (three large squares). Bazett's correction is therefore required. Three large squares= 3 x 0.2 seconds = 0.6 second. The R−R interval is 10 large squares = 10 x 0.2 second = 2 second. The Q−Tc is therefore:

$$\frac{0.6}{\sqrt{2}} = 0.42 \text{ second}$$

T waves

T waves are normal in size and shape.

Conclusion – third-degree heart block with a ventricular rate of 30 beats per minute. This rhythm is resulting in symptomatic hypotension. Consideration should be given to an emergency pacing procedure, followed by the placement of a permanent pacemaker.

The patient eventually had a permanent pacemaker inserted. An ECG was performed to check its function, and is shown below. Note the presence of pacing spikes, which indicate that the pacemaker is discharging. When a pacemaker stimulates the ventricles directly, the QRS complexes will be wide and bizarre. It is impossible to interpret anything else from the ECG in such circumstances, other than that an artificial pacemaker is present.

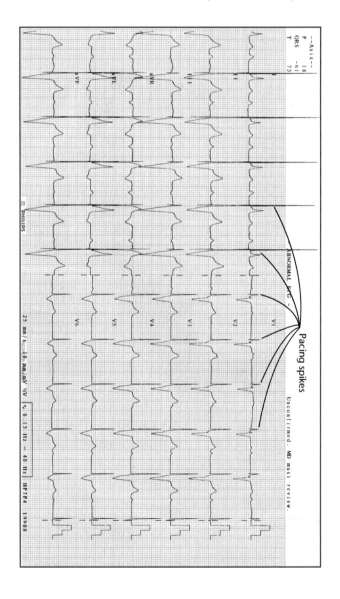

Pacing spikes

Case 76

A 52-year-old male shop assistant presents as an emergency to his general practitioner complaining of central chest pain. This has been present for 30 minutes. He is sweaty and short of breath, and complains of nausea. His risk factors for ischaemic heart disease include smoking and hypertension.

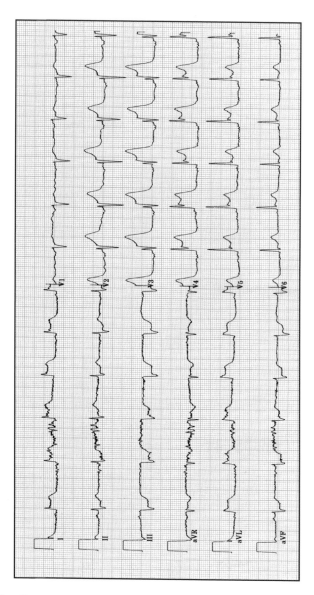

His ECG is shown. How would you interpret it?

Answer 76

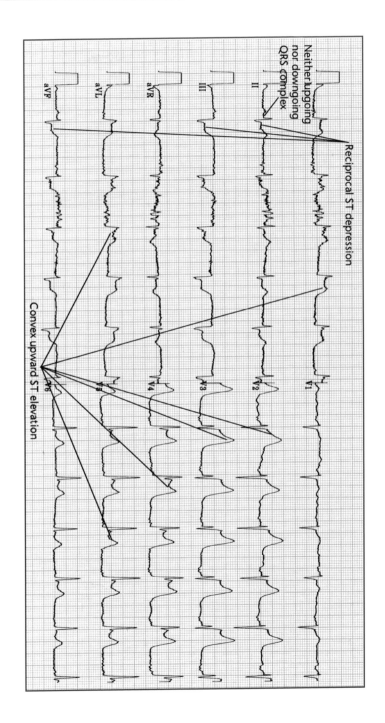

Heart rate

There are 4.2 big squares between consecutive R waves. The ventricular rate is therefore $300 \div 4.2 = 71$ beats per minute.

Heart rhythm

A P wave precedes each QRS complex. The P–R interval is normal (four small squares) and does not vary from beat to beat. The rhythm is sinus rhythm.

Cardiac axis

Lead I is upgoing. Lead III is downgoing. Lead II is neither upgoing nor downgoing. The axis is approaching that of left axis deviation.

P waves

P waves are of normal size and shape.

QRS complexes

There are no abnormal Q waves. The R and S waves are of normal height. The QRS complex is of normal duration (two small squares).

ST segment

The ST segment is elevated, in a convex shape, in leads I, aVL, V2, V3, V4 and V5. The ST segment is depressed and horizontal in leads II, III, aVR and aVF. When ST depression accompanies ST elevation, it is known as reciprocal ST depression.

QT interval

The QT interval is normal (1.5 large squares).

T waves

The T waves appear large, but are difficult to interpret on account of the ST segment changes.

Conclusion – anterolateral ST elevation myocardial infarction or STEMI (ie affecting the anterior and lateral surfaces of the heart). Reciprocal ST depression in some of the limb leads.

Case 77

An 80-year-old female nursing home resident presents with acute confusion. No other history is available. On examination, she is tachypnoeic, with oxygen saturations of 83% on 85% oxygen. She is peripherally cyanosed. Blood pressure is 74/32 mmHg. On auscultating her lungs, she has medium inspiratory crepitations to her midzones.

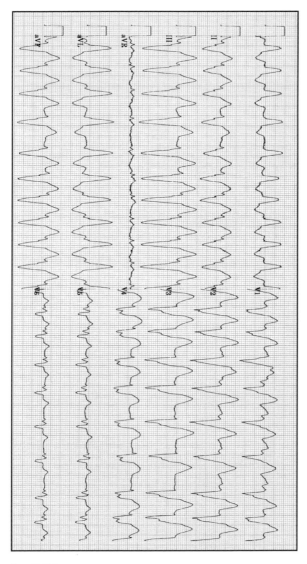

Interpret the ECG

Answer 77

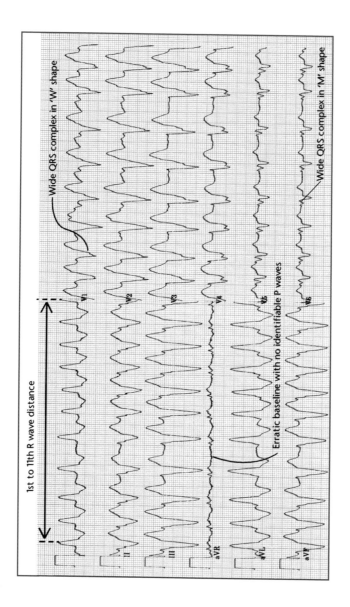

Heart rate

There are 11 small squares between the first 2 consecutive R waves in lead I. The ventricular rate is therefore $1500 \div 11 = 136$ beats per minute. However, since the rhythm is irregular, a more accurate assessment of heart rate can be made by measuring the distance between the first and eleventh R waves and dividing this distance by 10 to find the average R–R interval.

By this method, there are 24 large squares between the first and eleventh R waves. The average R–R interval is therefore 2.4 large squares. The heart rate is $300 \div 2.4 = 125$ beats per minute.

Heart rhythm

No P waves are visible. The baseline is erratic. QRS complexes occur irregularly. The rhythm is atrial fibrillation.

Cardiac axis

Lead I is upgoing. Leads II and III are downgoing. There is left axis deviation.

P waves

No P waves are visible.

QRS complexes

The QRS complexes are abnormally wide. The complex in V1 has a 'W' shape, and that in V6 is 'M' shaped. This is left bundle-branch block.

ST segment

The ST segment is difficult to visualise.

Q–T interval

The Q–T interval is difficult to measure.

T waves

T waves appear grossly abnormal in size and shape.

Conclusion – atrial fibrillation at 125 beats per minute with left bundle-branch block. When this pattern is present, it is impossible to make any further comments about an ECG (ie ST segment changes or T-wave abnormalities). Left bundle-branch block that is of new onset would be in keeping with an acute myocardial infarction. Old ECGs should be reviewed to determine whether this ECG finding is new.

Case 78

You are called to a cardiac arrest. Nursing staff have attached ECG electrodes, and the following rhythm is noted on the monitor. What is the rhythm?

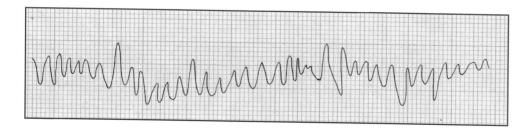

Answer 78

It is entirely possible to approach the interpretation of this rhythm as with all the ECGs above. However, for practical purposes, this rhythm should be instantly recognised as ventricular fibrillation (VF) by its erratic nature, and appropriate treatment given. This involves cardiac defibrillation.

After delivering three shocks, the rhythm on the monitor changes to that shown below. A pulse is still not present. What is the rhythm now?

Again, this strip can be analysed in detail, but it should be instantly recognised by its shape as ventricular tachycardia (VT). The ECG shows a tachycardia with wide QRS complexes. This rhythm can be associated with a cardiac output, so it would be imperative to check for the presence of a pulse. Cardiac arrest associated with VT is treated with defibrillation.

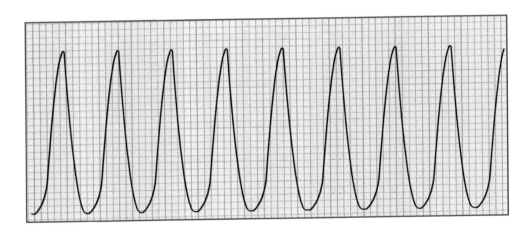

Echocardiography

It is unlikely that you will be required to have detailed knowledge of echocardiography at undergraduate level. However, it is important that you are familiar with echocardiographic reports and understand how to interpret them.

You may find it helpful to use the following headings when reading echocardiographic reports. Common abnormalities and points to bear in mind are also listed.

COMPONENT OF REPORT	COMMENT
Size of heart chambers (atria and ventricles)	The normal maximum diameter of the left atrium is 4.5 cm. The normal maximum diameter of the left ventricle in diastole is 5.5 cm
Ventricular septal thickness	This should be less than 1.2 cm. A thickened septum should raise suspicions of hypertrophic obstructive cardiomyopathy
Left ventricular function	Hypokinesis refers to walls that contract poorly. The left ventricular ejection fraction is normally around 65%
Details about each valve	Stenotic or regurgitant valves will often be described in terms of severity as trace, mild, moderate or severe. Often pressure gradients across valves and valve areas are documented. For the aortic valve, severe stenosis is present if there is a pressure gradient of more than 50 mmHg across the valve, or if the valve area is less than 1 cm^2
Vegetations or tumours	Bear in mind that a small vegetation may be missed with transthoracic echocardiography. Trans-oesophageal echocardiography is more reliable
Estimated pulmonary artery pressure	A pressure greater than 35 mmHg suggests pulmonary hypertension. Note that this is an estimated pressure reading only
Pericardial effusion	Present or absent

Case 79

A 67-year-old woman is reviewed in the cardiology clinic 2 months after a myocardial infarction. She complains of shortness of breath on walking 100 metres on the flat, which she did not have before her heart attack. On further questioning, she reports having to sleep on five pillows to prevent shortness of breath. An echocardiogram is requested.

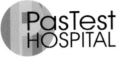

PasTest
HOSPITAL

Aortic root diameter is 3.3 cm

Morphologically normal aortic valve. No restriction of aortic valve leaflet opening. Aortic regurgitation (trace)

Left ventricular cavity size and wall thickness are normal. Left ventricular diastolic cavity diameter is 5.1 cm. Septal diastolic thickness is 1.1 cm

Posterior wall thickness is 1.1 cm. Severely hypokinetic anterior wall. Left ventricular ejection fraction is 25%

Morphologically normal mitral valve. Mitral regurgitation (trace)

Normal left atrial dimensions

Estimated pulmonary artery systolic pressure is 22 mmHg

Normal right ventricular cavity dimension. Right ventricular systolic function is normal. Normal tricuspid valve

Normal inferior vena cava and hepatic vein size indicating normal venous pressures

Technically fair study. Other cardiac valves and chambers appear normal. No pericardial effusion. No evidence of bacterial endocarditis on this study

How would you explain this woman's symptoms?

Answer 79

The important points to take away from the echocardiographic report are as follows:

Size of heart chambers (atria and ventricles)	Normal
Ventricular septal thickness	Normal
Left ventricular function	Severe left ventricular wall hypo-kinesis. Markedly reduced left ventricular ejection fraction
Details about each valve	Only a trace of aortic and mitral regurgitation
Vegetations or tumours	None seen
Estimated pulmonary artery pressure	Normal
Pericardial effusion	None

This woman has symptoms (dyspnoea and orthopnoea) of left ventricular failure. Her echocardiogram demonstrates the poor residual function of her left ventricle following her myocardial infarction.

Dynamic tests in cardiology

Exercise stress testing is commonly used to investigate ischaemic heart disease. In the resting state, a patient with significant coronary artery atherosclerosis may have a normal ECG. However, when the heart is put under stress by exercising, its energy requirements increase. If sufficient blood cannot be supplied to the myocardium under such circumstances, the tissue becomes ischaemic and the ECG will change. This is the basis of the exercise stress test.

ECG tracings are taken before, during and after exercise. Features that would be in keeping with ischaemic heart disease include horizontal or down-sloping ST segment depression or elevation, particularly if these are associated with angina or a reduction in blood pressure.

Other dynamic tests are used to assess cardiac function in particular patient groups. In patients who are unable to exercise, pharmacological agents (eg adenosine or dobutamine) can be administered to increase the heart rate and put the heart under stress. Cardiac function can then be assessed by performing echocardiography or by nuclear imaging techniques which look at the uptake of isotopes by cardiac muscle. By so-doing, areas of the heart that pump defectively or have inadequate blood supply can be identified.

PATHOLOGY

11

PATHOLOGY

This chapter lists typical pathological findings for a range of disease states. It is not by any means comprehensive, but includes most of the classic abnormalities that are commonly tested in general medical examinations. Further reading will be required when preparing for pathology examinations.

DISEASE	TYPICAL PATHOLOGICAL CHANGES
Gastroenterology	
Barrett's oesophagus	Lower oesophageal epithelium undergoes metaplasia to become gastric or intestinal-type epithelium
Coeliac disease	Total or subtotal villous atrophy in the small bowel Crypt hyperplasia with inflammatory cells in the mucosa
Crohn's disease	Can affect any part of the gastrointestinal tract *Macroscopically*: skip lesions (ie lengths of normal bowel between diseased segments); cobblestone appearance with fissured ulcers *Microscopically*: thickened wall with transmural inflammation; granulomata
Ulcerative colitis	Affects large bowel only Affects mucosa and submucosa only Crypt abscesses and superficial ulcers
Chronic cholecystitis	Chronic inflammatory changes Rokitansky–Aschoff sinuses
Hepatology	
Acute viral hepatitis	Swelling of hepatocytes with spotty necrosis Councilman's bodies

DISEASE	TYPICAL PATHOLOGICAL CHANGES
Alcoholic hepatitis	Fatty accumulation in cytoplasmic vacuoles, necrosis, Mallory's hyaline material
Chronic active hepatitis	Piecemeal necrosis
Autoimmune hepatitis	Interface hepatitis, portal plasma cell infiltration
Haemochromatosis	Excessive hepatic iron (shows up blue on Perls' stain)
Primary biliary cirrhosis	Portal hepatitis and granulomatous destruction of bile ducts. Later, periportal hepatitis and bile duct proliferation
Liver cirrhosis	*Macroscopically*: macronodular or micronodular *Microscopically*: fibrous tissue (shows up red on van Gieson's stain)

Respiratory

Diffuse alveolar damage (DAD) which can lead to adult respiratory distress syndrome (ARDS)	Alveolar hyaline membranes and thickened alveolar walls
Previous asbestos exposure	Asbestos bodies in lung
Pulmonary fibrosis	Proliferation of type II pneumocytes with thickening of the alveolar walls

Nephrology

Malignant hypertension	Renal arteriole fibrinoid necrosis
Diabetic glomerulosclerosis	Kimmelstiel–Wilson nodules, thickened capillary basement membranes with hyalinisation of arterioles

DISEASE	TYPICAL PATHOLOGICAL CHANGES
Haematology	
Hodgkin's disease	Reed–Sternberg cells Abnormal lymph node architecture Nodular sclerosing type has fibrous tissue
Myelofibrosis	Bone marrow fibrosis secondary to fibroblast pro-liferation
Multiple myeloma	Plasma cell proliferation in bone marrow
Rheumatology	
Temporal arteritis	Temporal artery biopsy may be normal Alternatively, plasma cells, lymphocytes and multinucleate giant cells can be present
Polymyositis	Muscle fibre necrosis Lymphocyte infiltration
Endocrinology	
Pituitary tumours	Acromegaly is associated with acidophil macroadenomas (somatotroph adenomas) Hyperprolactinaemia is associated with chromophobe adenomas ACTH excess is associated with basophil microadenomas (corticotroph adenomas)
Neurology	
Alzheimer's disease	*Macroscopically*: thinning of gyri *Microscopically*: neurofibrillary tangles; plaques
Parkinson's disease and dementia with Lewy bodies	Lewy bodies (inclusions inside neurons)
Obstetrics and gynaecology	
Ovarian endometriosis	*Macroscopically*: chocolate cyst

GENETICS

12

GENETICS

Family trees

In clinical practice, family trees are often recorded when there is a suspicion that a disease may have a familial element.

To the untrained eye, interpretation of family trees can seem like a daunting process, and many students resort to guessing what the inheritance pattern might be. However, if a few simple rules are borne in mind, interpretation can be made fairly simple. Being able to work out the expected inheritance patterns for the common mendelian disorders from first principles is a good way to check that your answer is correct.

Work through the various inheritance patterns for the common mendelian disorders below, and attempt to reproduce the information for yourself. This will be much easier to remember than if you simply learn off a list of rules.

The two main classes of conditions that are inherited in a mendelian manner are:

- autosomal conditions (affecting the autosomes, ie chromosomes 1 to 22)
- sex chromosomal conditions (affecting the sex chromosomes, ie X and Y).

Genotype refers to the genetic code
Phenotype refers to the actual manifestation of the genetic code

Autosomal conditions

Autosomal dominant inheritance

There are usually two copies of each chromosome in each cell, each carrying copies of the same genes. In autosomal dominant conditions, inheritance of one faulty gene is sufficient to give rise to the disorder. Thus one chromosome in the pair will be normal; the other will carry the faulty gene.

In the following diagram, the letter 'a' is used to denote a normal chromosome. The capital letter 'A' represents a chromosome with an abnormal gene. Thus an individual with two 'a' chromosomes will be normal. Someone with one 'a' chromosome and one 'A' chromosome will have the disorder, since only one faulty gene is needed for the condition to be manifest. If both parents are affected, it would also be possible for offspring to have two 'A' chromosomes.

Since 50% of the offspring's genetic code comes from one parent and 50% from the other, there is a 50% chance that either chromosome will be passed on.

		Mother	
		a	a
	a	aa	aa
Father			
	A	Aa	Aa

In the example, the father has an autosomal dominant condition, and therefore has one normal chromosome (a) and one abnormal chromosome (A). The mother has two normal chromosomes. There are four possible ways that the genes can be passed onto the offspring (aa, aa, Aa and Aa).

Thus for autosomal dominant conditions:

- both males and females can be affected
- if one parent is affected, there will be a 50% chance that a child will also be affected.

Autosomal recessive inheritance

For an autosomal recessive disorder to be manifest, both chromosomes in a pair must carry the abnormal gene. One abnormal gene must therefore be passed on from each parent.

If a person has one normal and one abnormal chromosome, he or she is a termed 'a carrier' and does not exhibit any features of the disorder, and therefore will appear normal (ie normal phenotype).

The inheritance pattern for one carrier parent and one normal parent will be as follows (remember 'a' is the normal chromosome, and 'A' the abnormal).

		Mother	
		a	a
	a	aa	aa
Father			
	A	Aa	Aa

For autosomal recessive conditions with one carrier parent:

- both male and female offspring can be carriers
- 50% of the offspring will be carriers.

The inheritance pattern for two carrier parents will be as follows.

	Mother	
	a	A
a	aa	aA
A	Aa	AA

Father

For autosomal recessive conditions with two carrier parents:

- both male and female offspring can be carriers or be affected
- 50% of the offspring will be carriers
- 25% of the offspring will be normal (ie not carriers)
- 25% of the offspring will have the condition.

The inheritance pattern for one affected parent will be as follows.

	Mother	
	a	a
A	Aa	Aa
A	Aa	Aa

Father

For autosomal recessive conditions with an affected parent:

- both male and female offspring can be carriers
- all offspring will be carriers.

Sex chromosomal conditions

X-linked recessive inheritance

X-linked disorders involve faulty genes found on the X chromosome. Since females have two X chromosomes, having one faulty chromosome is of minor consequence with a recessive disorder, because the other X chromosome is normal. Males, however, have only one X (but also one Y) chromosome. A faulty X chromosome in a male will therefore result in phenotypical effects.

If a female has one abnormal X chromosome, they are termed 'a carrier' and generally do not exhibit any features of the disorder. Occasionally mild signs of disease may be present.

The inheritance pattern for a carrier mother and a normal father will be as follows (X = normal chromosome, X = abnormal chromosome):

		Mother	
		X	X
	X	XX	XX
Father			
	Y	YX	YX

For X-linked recessive disorders with a carrier mother:

- only males can be affected
- 50% of male offspring will have the disorder
- 50% of female offspring will be carriers
- 50% of all offspring will be normal.

The inheritance pattern for an affected father and a normal mother will be as follows:

		Mother	
		X	X
	X	XX	XX
Father			
	Y	YX	YX

For X-linked recessive disorders with an affected father:

- no offspring will be affected
- all daughters will be carriers
- all sons will be normal.

X-linked dominant inheritance

In these disorders, only one faulty X chromosome is necessary for the disease to be manifest. Thus, diseases can occur in both male and females.

The inheritance pattern for an affected mother and a normal father will be as follows:

		Mother	
		X	X
Father	X	XX	XX
	Y	YX	YX

For X-linked dominant disorders with an affected mother:

- both males and females can be affected
- 50% of male offspring will have the disorder
- 50% of female offspring will have the disorder.

The inheritance pattern for an affected father and a normal mother will be as follows:

		Mother	
		X	X
Father	X	XX	XX
	Y	YX	YX

For X-linked dominant disorders with an affected father:

- only female offspring can be affected
- all daughters will have the disorder
- all sons will be normal.

Other modes of inheritance

Mitochondrial inheritance

Mitochondria are cellular organelles that have a major role in energy production. They have their own DNA, which may undergo mutations. Diseases caused by mitochondrial genetic problems have an interesting inheritance pattern resulting from the fact that female ova all contain mitochondria, however male sperm do not. Therefore, mitochondrial disorders can be passed on only by females. To summarise:

- both males and females can be affected

- affected females can pass on the disorder to all offspring

- affected males cannot pass on the disorder.

Genetic imprinting

This phenomenon relates to the fact that certain genes are expressed only if inherited from a particular parent. This can best be explained by looking at two conditions – Prader–Willi and Angelman syndromes. For Prader–Willi syndrome, only the paternal gene is important. Failure to inherit the paternal copy will therefore result in the syndrome. Angelman syndrome results from failure to inherit the maternal gene. The disorders may result from gene deletion mutations, where the gene from a particular parent is deleted. Alternatively, they may arise when two chromosomes are inherited from one parent rather than one from each. This is known as uniparental disomy.

> **MEMORY AID**
>
> In **P**rader–Willi syndrome – the **P**aternal gene is inactive
> In Angel**m**an syndrome – the **M**aternal gene is inactive

Other points

Variable expression relates to the fact that a person may carry the necessary genetic make-up for a condition, but not exhibit all the phenotypical features. At the extreme of this is 'non-penetrance' where the person has no features of the condition.

Genetic disorders may appear to arise out of the blue, with no family members being affected. This is most commonly due to a new genetic mutation, but can also result from gonadal mosaicism where a parent carries the mutated genes only in the germ cells.

Family tree interpretation

When faced with a family tree, and asked to comment on inheritance patterns, the flow diagram below should be helpful.

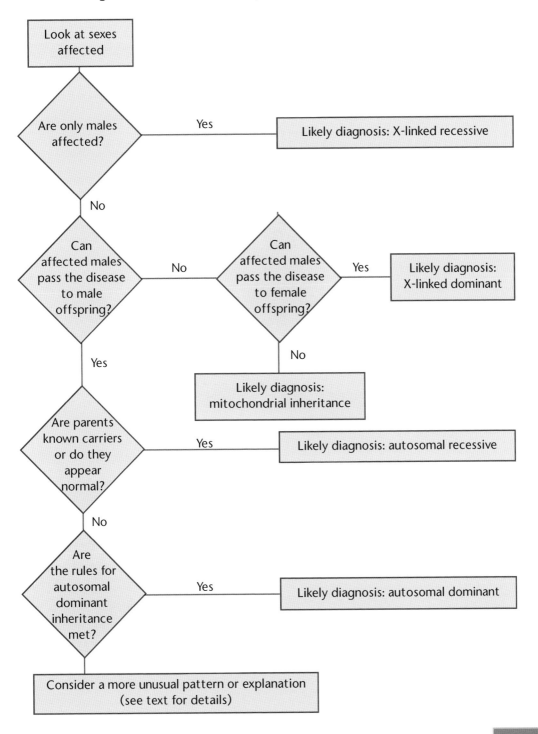

Examples of genetic conditions with different inheritance patterns

Those most commonly tested in undergraduate examinations are highlighted in bold in the following table.

MODE OF INHERITANCE	EXAMPLES
Autosomal dominant	Achondroplasia **Adult polycystic kidney disease** **Dystrophia myotonica** Ehlers–Danlos syndrome Familial adenomatous polyposis **Familial hypercholesterolaemia** Hereditary haemorrhagic telangiectasia **Huntington's disease** **Marfan's syndrome** **Neurofibromatosis** Noonan's syndrome Osteogenesis imperfecta Otosclerosis **Tuberous sclerosis**
Autosomal recessive	Albinism Congenital adrenal hyperplasia **Cystic fibrosis** Friedreich's ataxia Galactosaemia Glycogen storage diseases **Hereditary haemochromatosis** Hurler's syndrome Oculocutaneous albinism Phenylketonuria **Sickle cell disease** Tay–Sachs disease Thalassaemia Wilson's disease
X-linked dominant	Vitamin-D-resistant rickets

X-linked recessive	Alport's syndrome
	Becker's muscular dystrophy
	Duchenne muscular dystrophy
	Fragile X syndrome
	Glucose-6-phosphate dehydrogenase deficiency
	Haemophilia A
	Haemophilia B
	Hunter's syndrome
Mitochondrial	Leber-hereditary optic neuropathy

Karyotype analysis

The following table lists the common chromosomal abnormalities that you would be expected to recognise.

CHROMOSOMAL ABNORMALITY	CONDITION
Trisomy 21	Down's syndrome
Trisomy 18	Edwards' syndrome
Trisomy 12	Patau's syndrome
45, XO	Turner's syndrome
47, XXY	Klinefelter's syndrome
47, XXX	Triple X syndrome
47, XXY	Associated with behavioural problems
5p−	Cri-du-chat syndrome
Microdeletion at 22q11	DiGeorge syndrome
Microdeletion at 7q11	Williams's syndrome

Common mutations

DISEASE	COMMON MUTATION
Cystic fibrosis	ΔF508 mutation on long arm of chromosome 7. This codes for the cystic fibrosis transmembrane conductance regulator
Haemochromatosis	C282Y mutation on the *HFE* gene on the short arm of chromosome 6. The H63D mutation can also be found

Case 80

What is the inheritance pattern in the following family tree?

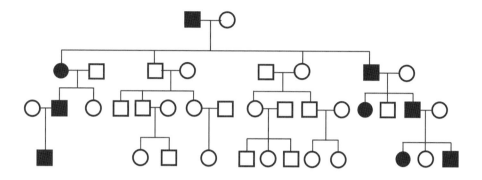

Key

▢ unaffected male   ■ affected male

◯ unaffected female   ● affected female

Answer 80

- Both males and females are affected
- Male-to-male inheritance is possible
- One of the parents of all affected cases is also affected.
- If one parent is affected, there appears to be approximately a 50% chance that a child will also be affected.

The inheritance pattern is therefore autosomal dominant.

Case 81

Some members of the following family suffer from a rare bone disease. What is the inheritance pattern?

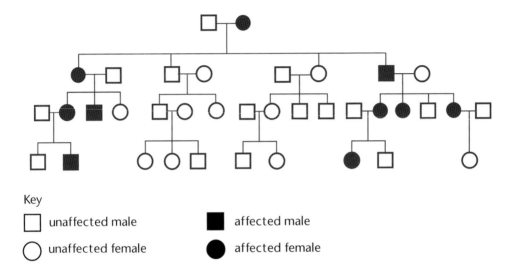

Key

☐	unaffected male	■	affected male
○	unaffected female	●	affected female

Answer 81

- Both males and females are affected
- There are no instances of male-to-male transmission
- Male-to-female transmission is possible, with all daughters of an affected male having the condition.

The likely diagnosis is vitamin-D-resistant rickets, with the inheritance pattern being X-linked dominant.

Case 82

Some family members have a rare genetic disorder. This is their family tree. What is the likely inheritance pattern?

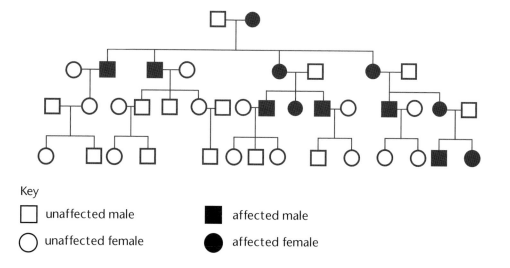

Key

☐ unaffected male   ■ affected male

○ unaffected female   ● affected female

Answer 82

- Both males and females are affected
- Male-to-male and male-to-female transmission do not occur
- Affected females pass the condition on to all offspring.

The inheritance pattern is mitochondrial.

RESPIRATORY MEDICINE

13

RESPIRATORY MEDICINE

Arterial blood gas analysis

Arterial blood gas (ABG) analysis provides a wealth of information about a patient's state of health. The test is most commonly used in acute illness but may also be used in the assessment of patients with chronic respiratory disease. In acute situations, multiple analyses are often made to assess response to treatment. Trends are usually more helpful than one-off readings. Never forget to consult old medical records if possible, since the patient's baseline may be well outside 'normal' limits.

Interpretation of four key indices – pH, partial pressure of oxygen (PaO_2), partial pressure of carbon dioxide ($PaCO_2$) and bicarbonate (HCO_3^-) – will provide most of the information needed in clinical practice. A fifth index, base excess, can also be used, but will not be discussed here in detail.

Sophisticated blood gas analysers will provide other useful information such as blood levels of lactate and methaemoglobin.

NORMAL RANGES (BREATHING ROOM AIR AT SEA LEVEL)

pH	7.35–7.45
PaO_2	11–13 kPa
$PaCO_2$	4.7–6.0 kPa
HCO_3^-	24–30 mmol/l
Base excess	−2 to +2 mmol/l
Anion gap	12–16 mmol/l

Systematic interpretation of an ABG

Assess oxygenation

You will note that the normal range for PaO_2 given in the box above was 11–13 kPa. This value holds true for a patient breathing room air that contains 21% oxygen. It is crucial to appreciate that a patient with normal lungs will have a much higher PaO_2 if their inspired oxygen concentration (FiO_2) is increased. The physiology behind this is summarised in the alveolar gas equation, which is beyond the scope of this book. For day-to-day practice, the information in the following box should help detect any major problems.

INSPIRED OXYGEN CONCENTRATION (%)	EXPECTED PaO_2 WITH HEALTHY LUNGS (kPa)
28	21
35	27
40	32
60	51
85	75
100	89

MEMORY AID

As a rule of thumb, the expected PaO_2 (in kPa) is roughly 10 less than the FiO_2 (in %)

It is therefore impossible to interpret the PaO2 without knowing the FiO_2. If the PaO_2 is lower than expected, this implies that a disease process in the lungs is interfering with gas exchange. This can occur with a variety of conditions, such as pulmonary oedema or pneumonia.

DON'T FORGET

Always interpret the PaO_2 with the FiO_2 in mind

With the above in mind, decide whether oxygenation is normal or abnormal.

The label of 'respiratory failure' is used when the PaO_2 is less than 8 kPa. It is divided into two types depending on the $PaCO_2$, as follows:

RESPIRATORY FAILURE TYPE	PaO_2 (kPa)	$PaCO_2$ (kPa)
Type 1	<8	<6.5
Type 2	<8	>6.5

MEMORY AID

In type **ONE** respiratory failure, **ONE** gas is abnormal (ie low O_2, without high CO_2)
In type **TWO** respiratory failure, **TWO** gases are abnormal (both O_2 and CO_2)

COMMON CAUSES OF RESPIRATORY FAILURE

TYPE 1	TYPE 2
Pulmonary oedema	Chronic obstructive pulmonary disease
Pneumonia	(COPD) — blue bloaters
Pulmonary embolism	Respiratory centre depression
Pulmonary fibrosis	Respiratory muscle weakness
COPD – pink puffers	Abnormal chest wall

Assess acid–base status

Look at the pH

Is it:

- normal (7.35–7.45)

- low (<7.35) indicating acidosis

- high (>7.45) indicating alkalosis

Look at the $PaCO_2$

Is it normal, low or high? Carbon dioxide is an acidic gas, so, with high levels in the system, one would expect an acidosis. Similarly, with low levels, an alkalosis is expected.

Look at the HCO_3^-

Is it normal, low or high? Bicarbonate is alkaline. High levels should therefore be associated with an alkalosis, low levels an acidosis.

Put these three parts together using the following flow chart. You may find it useful to try to memorise the flow chart initially, but with practice it will become intuitive.

Fig 13.1: Interpretation of common arterial blood gas abnormalities

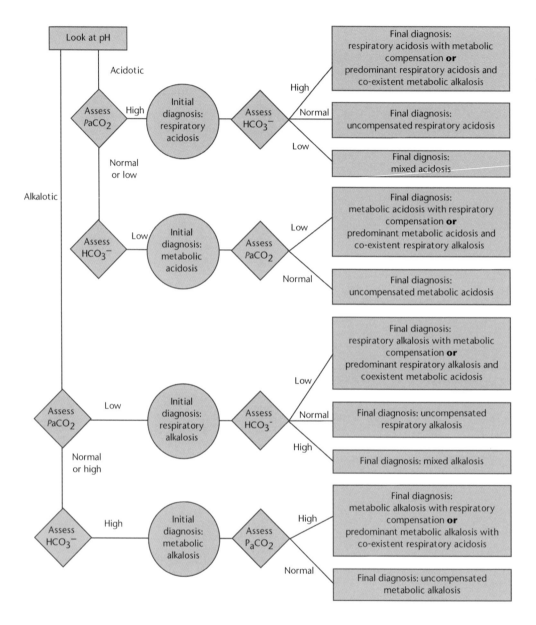

Respiratory acidosis can be due to any of the causes of respiratory failure.

Respiratory alkalosis is always due to hyperventilation. Be wary of attributing hyperventilation exclusively to anxiety, however, since it may occur secondary to an underlying severe disease process, such as sepsis or stroke.

There are a wide range of causes for a metabolic acidosis. To narrow down this list, and help you come to a diagnosis, it is helpful to calculate the anion gap. If this is high (>16 mmol/l), the acidosis is due to the presence of excess acids in the body that are not routinely analysed in the laboratory. The anion gap is calculated as follows:

$$\text{Anion gap} = (Na^+ + K^+) - (Cl^- + HCO_3^-)$$

A patient with the following biochemical findings — Na^+ 136 mmol/l, K^+ 3.5 mmol/l, Cl^- 100 mmol/l, HCO_3^- 24 mmol/l — would therefore have an anion gap of 15.5 mmol/l.

DON'T FORGET

Always calculate the anion gap in a patient with a metabolic acidosis

---

COMMON CAUSES OF A METABOLIC ACIDOSIS

NORMAL ANION GAP	RAISED ANION GAP
HCO_3^- loss from gut, eg diarrhoea	Ketoacidosis
Renal tubular acidosis	Renal failure
	Lactic acidosis
	Salicylate toxicity
	Methanol ingestion
	Ethylene glycol (antifreeze) ingestion

COMMON CAUSES OF A METABOLIC ALKALOSIS

Losses from the gut, particularly vomiting (classically pyloric stenosis)
Primary or secondary hyperaldosteronism
Hypercalcaemia
Use of diuretics
Bicarbonate ingestion

> **DON'T FORGET**
>
> A normal pH with an abnormal $PaCO_2$ or HCO_3^- indicates complete compensation

The seven ABG abnormalities that you might be asked to interpret are:

1. Type 1 respiratory failure
2. Type 2 respiratory failure
3. Respiratory acidosis
4. Respiratory alkalosis
5. Metabolic acidosis with a normal anion gap
6. Metabolic acidosis with a raised anion gap
7. Metabolic alkalosis.

Note that the first two are problems primarily with oxygenation that might co-exist with an acid–base disturbance.

Abnormalities 3–7 may all occur with compensation.

Case 83

The blood gas below was taken following admission of an elderly patient to the acute medical unit. He was breathing room air.

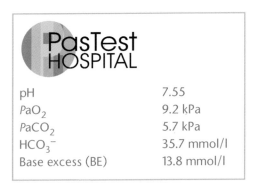

PasTest
HOSPITAL

pH	7.55
PaO_2	9.2 kPa
$PaCO_2$	5.7 kPa
HCO_3^-	35.7 mmol/l
Base excess (BE)	13.8 mmol/l

1. **Outline the abnormalities on this ABG.**

2. **What are the likely causes for these abnormalities?**

Answer 83

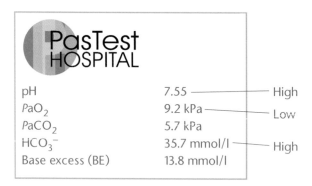

PasTest
HOSPITAL

pH	7.55	High
PaO_2	9.2 kPa	Low
$PaCO_2$	5.7 kPa	
HCO_3^-	35.7 mmol/l	High
Base excess (BE)	13.8 mmol/l	

1. Oxygenation is abnormal, ie the PaO_2 is lower than normal for a patient breathing room air.

   The pH is high, indicating an alkalosis. The $PaCO_2$ is normal, and the HCO_3^- is high. Using the flow diagram on page 312, you can work out that this represents an uncompensated metabolic alkalosis.

2. Poor oxygenation could reflect any disease process affecting the lungs. Common causes would be pulmonary oedema or pneumonia.
   The causes of a metabolic alkalosis are listed in the box on page 313.
   The patient in this case had a lower respiratory tract infection and vomiting.

Case 84

A 68-year-old man with a 40-pack-year smoking history was admitted short of breath and with a cough productive of green sputum. On examination he was tachypnoeic and using his accessory muscles of respiration. Auscultation of his chest revealed widespread expiratory wheeze with bibasal coarse crepitations. He was placed on 28% oxygen and his initial ABG is shown below.

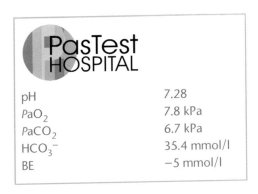

PasTest HOSPITAL	
pH	7.28
PaO_2	7.8 kPa
$PaCO_2$	6.7 kPa
HCO_3^-	35.4 mmol/l
BE	−5 mmol/l

1. **Outline the abnormalities on this ABG.**

2. **What is the likely diagnosis?**

3. **What type of assisted ventilation could be considered in the management of this condition?**

Answer 84

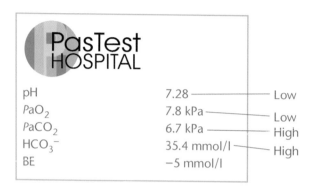

PasTest HOSPITAL		
pH	7.28	Low
PaO₂	7.8 kPa	Low
PaCO₂	6.7 kPa	High
HCO₃⁻	35.4 mmol/l	High
BE	−5 mmol/l	

1. Oxygenation is abnormal. The patient has type 2 respiratory failure, with low PaO_2 and high $PaCO_2$.

   The pH is low, indicating an acidosis. The $PaCO_2$ is high, as is the HCO_3^-. Using the flow chart you can see that this pattern could represent either respiratory acidosis with metabolic compensation, or a predominant respiratory acidosis with a coexistent metabolic alkalosis.

2. The most likely diagnosis is an acute exacerbation of chronic obstructive pulmonary disease (COPD). This would be in keeping with the clinical findings. The acid–base disturbance would therefore represent respiratory acidosis with metabolic compensation. Note that the compensation is only partial, since the patient remains acidotic. An acute exacerbation of COPD is the commonest cause of a respiratory acidosis with a raised HCO_3^-.

   Many patients with COPD have high resting CO_2 levels, causing a respiratory acidosis. However, with time, the kidneys compensate for this acidosis by retaining HCO_3^-. Thus, in the 'normal' state, many patients with COPD have a normal pH, with a raised $PaCO_2$ and a raised HCO_3^-, such as that shown in the ABG below:

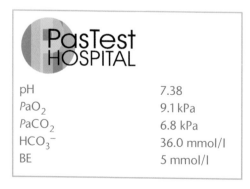

PasTest HOSPITAL	
pH	7.38
PaO₂	9.1 kPa
PaCO₂	6.8 kPa
HCO₃⁻	36.0 mmol/l
BE	5 mmol/l

During an acute exacerbation, however, the $PaCO_2$ levels increase, giving rise to a respiratory acidosis.

3. Patients may often benefit from non-invasive ventilation (NIV) using bi-level positive airway pressure (BiPAP). If deterioration occurs, intubation and ventilation may be required.

Case 85

An anxious 27-year-old student was admitted with shortness of breath and tingling in her hands. On examination, she had a respiratory rate of 28 breaths per minute. Chest examination was unremarkable. Chest X-ray and routine blood tests were normal. An ECG showed sinus tachycardia. An ABG was taken on 35% oxygen.

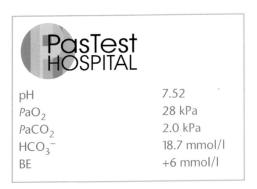

PasTest
HOSPITAL

pH	7.52
PaO_2	28 kPa
$PaCO_2$	2.0 kPa
HCO_3^-	18.7 mmol/l
BE	+6 mmol/l

1. **Outline the abnormalities on this ABG.**

2. **What is the likely cause?**

3. **How might one treat this woman?**

Answer 85

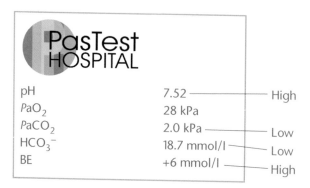

PasTest
HOSPITAL

pH	7.52	High
PaO$_2$	28 kPa	
PaCO$_2$	2.0 kPa	Low
HCO$_3^-$	18.7 mmol/l	Low
BE	+6 mmol/l	High

1. Oxygenation is normal given that the FiO_2 is 35%.
   The pH is high indicating an alkalosis. The $PaCO_2$ and HCO_3^- are both low.
   Using the flow chart, you can see that this pattern could be due to either a
   respiratory alkalosis with metabolic compensation or a predominant
   respiratory alkalosis with coexistent metabolic acidosis.

2. The likely cause for this ABG given the clinical history is hyperventilation.
   Thus the acid–base disturbance is a respiratory alkalosis with metabolic
   compensation. One of the commonest causes is anxiety, but it may occur as
   a result of organic pathology such as a stroke or subarachnoid haemorrhage
   affecting the respiratory centre.
   A full history and examination would be essential to help rule out a serious
   cause of this acid–base disturbance.

3. Reassurance would be a key aspect of treatment in the case of anxiety. Re-
   breathing one's own exhaled air, using a paper bag, may also be beneficial.

Case 86

A 32-year-old French tourist is brought to A&E feeling generally unwell. No history is available. He appears dehydrated and has a respiratory rate of 22 breaths per minute. The following ABG and biochemical profile are taken on admission, breathing room air.

PasTest
HOSPITAL

pH	7.26
PaO_2	11.5 kPa
$PaCO_2$	2.9 kPa
HCO_3^-	12.6 mmol/l
BE	−15.8 mmol/l
Na^+	131 mmol/l
K^+	4.5 mmol/l
Urea	8.8 mmol/l
Creatinine	130 µmol/l
Cl^-	96.1 mmol/l
HCO_3^-	15 mmol/l

METABOLIC ACIDOSIS
∴ CALC ANION GAP

$AG = (131 + 4.5) - (96.1 + 15)$
$135.5 - 111.1$
$= 26.8$
∴ Raised

1. **Outline the abnormalities seen.**

2. **What tests should you request?**

3. **Which drugs or substances taken in overdose could give a similar pattern?**

Answer 86

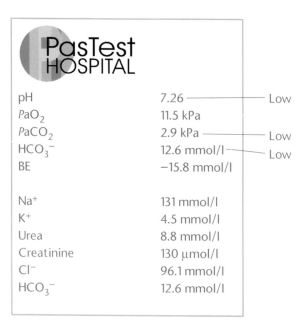

PasTest
HOSPITAL

pH	7.26	Low
PaO_2	11.5 kPa	
$PaCO_2$	2.9 kPa	Low
HCO_3^-	12.6 mmol/l	Low
BE	−15.8 mmol/l	
Na^+	131 mmol/l	
K^+	4.5 mmol/l	
Urea	8.8 mmol/l	
Creatinine	130 μmol/l	
Cl^-	96.1 mmol/l	
HCO_3^-	12.6 mmol/l	

1. Oxygenation is normal.
   The pH is low indicating an acidosis. The $PaCO_2$ and HCO_3^- are both low.
   Using the flow chart you can see that this indicates either a metabolic
   acidosis with respiratory compensation or a predominant metabolic acidosis
   with coexistent respiratory alkalosis.
   Remember to calculate the anion gap with any case of metabolic acidosis.
   In this case the anion gap is calculated as follows: $(131 + 4.5) - (96.1 + 12.6)$
   $= 26.8$. Thus this is a raised anion gap metabolic acidosis.

2. Bearing in mind the causes of a raised anion gap metabolic acidosis shown in
   the box on page 313, the following tests would be helpful: urinalysis for
   ketones, plasma lactate levels and salicylate levels.

3. This pattern can be seen when salicylates (eg aspirin), methanol or ethylene
   glycol is taken in excess.

Case 87

A 57-year-old man is medically retired from his former job in the local shipyard. For the past 6 years his health has deteriorated with an exercise tolerance now reduced to 10 metres on the flat. He is a life-long non-smoker. A recent high-resolution CT (HRCT) scan of the chest demonstrated diffuse bibasal interstitial changes. His ABG was taken on room air without any intercurrent illness.

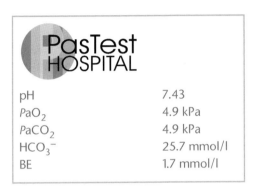

PasTest HOSPITAL	
pH	7.43
PaO_2	4.9 kPa
$PaCO_2$	4.9 kPa
HCO_3^-	25.7 mmol/l
BE	1.7 mmol/l

1. **Outline the abnormalities seen.**

2. **What are the likely causes for an ABG such as this?**

3. **What long-term therapy might be considered?**

Answer 87

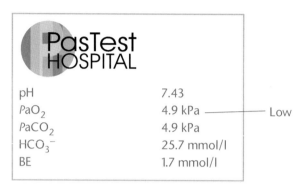

pH	7.43
PaO_2	4.9 kPa ——— Low
$PaCO_2$	4.9 kPa
HCO_3^-	25.7 mmol/l
BE	1.7 mmol/l

1. Oxygenation is abnormal. The patient has type 1 respiratory failure, with a low PaO_2 and normal $PaCO_2$.
   The pH is normal, as is the HCO_3^-.

2. This man's clinical history when taken in conjunction with his clinical signs and ABG is highly suggestive of pulmonary fibrosis. The fact that he worked in a shipyard may suggest exposure to asbestos, which is a potential cause of pulmonary fibrosis – especially at the lung bases as the CT scan suggests. Other causes for type 1 respiratory failure are listed in the box on page 311.

3. Long-term oxygen therapy (LTOT) could be considered. However, there are strict guidelines that must be met before LTOT is commenced.

Pulmonary function tests

Peak expiratory flow rate

Peak expiratory flow rate (PEFR) is a simple bedside test that gives a useful insight into the respiratory function of a patient. The PEFR is measured in litres per minute using a basic plastic device. An average recording of three attempts is documented on a peak flow chart. The trend in PEFR and its relationship to symptoms are a guide to the severity of illness and the effectiveness of treatment.

Some patients with asthma will keep records of their PEFR. For comparative purposes recordings should be taken at the same time each day. This will eliminate changes due to normal diurnal variation. There is a normal variation in PEFR in people with asthma, with a typical dip first thing in the morning.

It is important to appreciate when interpreting values that the normal PEFR varies with age, height and sex.

PATIENT	HEIGHT (cm)	NORMAL PEFR (l/min)
25-year-old male	175	630
25-year-old female	175	505
60-year-old male	160	545
60-year-old female	160	445

DON'T FORGET

PEFR varies with age, sex and height

Spirometry

Spirometry provides a wealth of information about lung volumes and function. Spirometry reports can appear confusing. However, by looking at four indices, most of the important patterns of lung disease can be distinguished.

KEY RESULTS IN SPIROMETRY		
INDEX	**ABBREVIATION**	**INTERPRETATION**
Forced expiratory volume in 1 second	FEV_1	The volume of air that can be expired in 1 second
Forced vital capacity	FVC	The volume of air expired in a complete expiration
Ratio of FEV_1 to FVC	FEV_1/FVC	—
Carbon monoxide transfer coefficient	K_{CO}	A measure of the rate of diffusion of carbon monoxide from the alveoli into the capillary blood

Values obtained by spirometry should always be compared with age and sex-matched control values. Often results are converted into percentages of the predicted value in order to simplify interpretation.

Arguably the most useful index is the FEV_1/FVC. This test can be used to distinguish between obstructive airway disease (eg asthma, chronic obstructive pulmonary disease [COPD]) and restrictive lung disease (eg pulmonary fibrosis). In an obstructive defect, the FEV_1/FVC will be less than 70%. The percentage is greater than 80% with a restrictive defect.

COMMON PATTERNS OF FEV_1/FVC
<70% in obstructive airway disease
>80% in restrictive lung disease

The theory underlying these patterns is easily understood. In a patient with obstructive airway disease, airway obstruction makes expiration slow (and usually wheezy). The FEV_1 is therefore typically low, since only a small volume of air can be expired in 1 second. These patients also 'trap air' so the FVC will usually be high. A low FEV_1 and a high FVC combine to give a low FEV_1/FVC. In other words, the volume of air in the lungs is normal or high, but it is not easily forced out.

In restrictive lung disease, on the other hand, there is no airway obstruction. The FEV_1 is therefore typically higher than with an obstructive defect (although it is still usually reduced compared with normal). Small lung volumes contribute to a low FVC. A relatively high FEV_1 and a low FVC combine to give a high FEV_1/FVC. Put simply, the patient can force air out of their lungs, but since the lung volume is reduced, there is less of it to force out.

The three main patterns of lung function (normal, obstructive and restrictive) are shown pictorially on the following chart.

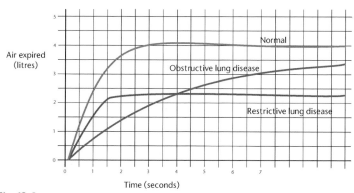

Fig 13.2

The K_{CO} measures the ease of diffusion of carbon monoxide from alveolar air to capillary blood. Anything that hinders gas transfer from alveolus into blood will therefore result in a low K_{CO}. Common causes of low K_{CO} are shown in the box below.

CAUSES OF A LOW K_{CO}

Interstitial lung disease
Emphysema
Pulmonary oedema
Pulmonary embolism
Anaemia

In rare cases, the K_{CO} can be raised. In such circumstances, gas transfers more easily than normal from alveolus into blood. Examples include polycythaemia (see Chapter 1, Haematology) or in cases of pulmonary haemorrhage (for example Goodpasture's syndrome).

Note that anaemia is the classic case where a patient will have a low K_{CO} with normal spirometry. The K_{CO} is low because there is less haemoglobin present to carry gas away from the alveoli.

Case 88

The following chart plots changes in PEFR of a patient with asthma during her hospital stay.

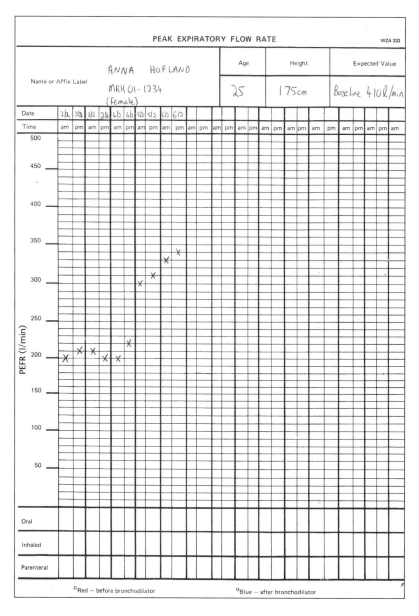

How would you interpret this chart?

Answer 88

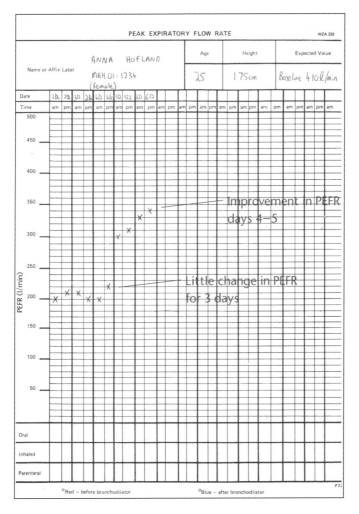

PEAK EXPIRATORY FLOW RATE

WZA 333

ANNA HOFLAND

MRH 01-1234
(Female)

Name or Affix Label

Age	Height	Expected Value
25	175cm	Baseline 410 l/min

Improvement in PEFR days 4–5

Little change in PEFR for 3 days

PEFR (l/min)

Oral

Inhaled

Parenteral

°Red – before bronchodilator   °Blue – after bronchodilator

In this bedside chart, the patient's known baseline PEFR of 410 l/min has been documented. Using the patient details at the top of the chart, one can look up the predicted PEFR, which is 505 l/min. Thus, even when at 'her best' she has a reduction in expiratory flow compared with a 'normal' adult of the same build. At the time of admission her PEFR is only 200 l/min – less than half of her baseline. Over the course of the next 2 days there is little change in her PEFR. Her condition has stabilised. Days 4 and 5 of her stay show a significant and sustained increase in her readings. A steady rise to 340 l/min is seen. There has either been a natural resolution of her asthma attack or the instigation of effective treatment has caused this change.

Case 89

A 70-year-old man with a long history of rheumatoid disease is reviewed at clinic. He complains that he is unable to make it to the newsagents any longer without having to stop to catch his breath. He has no history of chest or cardiovascular disease. He has no other symptoms. On examination, fine end-inspiratory crepitations are heard at both lung bases. Spirometry is requested.

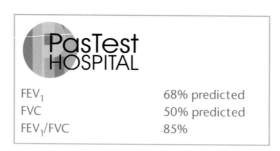

PasTest HOSPITAL	
FEV$_1$	68% predicted
FVC	50% predicted
FEV$_1$/FVC	85%

1. **Outline the abnormal findings in the results above.**

2. **What is the most likely cause for these abnormalities in this patient?**

3. **What imaging test would be most useful here?**

Answer 89

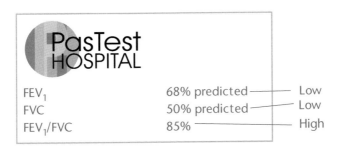

PasTest HOSPITAL		
FEV$_1$	68% predicted	Low
FVC	50% predicted	Low
FEV$_1$/FVC	85%	High

1. This man has a restrictive defect on spirometry as shown by the raised FEV$_1$/FVC.

2. The most likely cause would be pulmonary fibrosis, secondary to either his rheumatoid disease or as a side-effect of its treatment with methotrexate.

3. A HRCT scan of the chest would best aid diagnosis and management. This would identify any pulmonary changes associated with fibrosis.

Case 90

A 68-year-old man who has been a life-long smoker is admitted with a lower respiratory tract infection. He was noted to be wheezy at the time of admission to hospital, and was treated with antibiotics and nebulised bronchodilators. His inflammatory markers settled, but he remained wheezy. Pulmonary function tests were performed 3 weeks later after resolution of his acute illness.

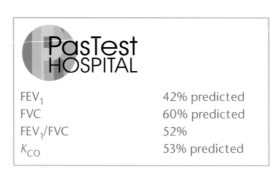

FEV$_1$	42% predicted
FVC	60% predicted
FEV$_1$/FVC	52%
K_{CO}	53% predicted

1. **Outline the abnormal findings in the results above.**

2. **What is the most likely cause for these abnormalities in this patient?**

Answer 90

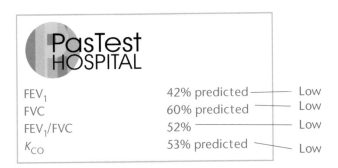

FEV$_1$	42% predicted	Low
FVC	60% predicted	Low
FEV$_1$/FVC	52%	Low
K_{CO}	53% predicted	Low

1. This patient's spirometry shows an obstructive pattern. His K_{CO} is low, indicating that something is interfering with gas transfer in the lungs. In this case, it is a reflection of his airway disease.

2. Given that this patient is a life-long smoker, it is likely that he has COPD. Consideration should be given to optimising inhaled bronchodilator therapy before discharge.

Case 91

A 64-year-old woman is admitted from A&E complaining of increasing shortness of breath. This has been increasing over a period of 2 months. There is little of note on examination. The admitting doctor arranges for pulmonary function tests to assess her symptom.

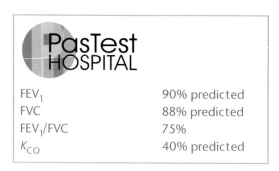

FEV_1	90% predicted
FVC	88% predicted
FEV_1/FVC	75%
K_{CO}	40% predicted

1. **Outline the abnormal findings in the results above.**

2. **What blood test would you order?**

Answer 91

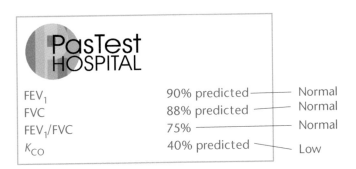

1. FEV$_1$ and FVC are considered normal unless they are less than 80% of the predicted value. Spirometry is essentially normal in this example. The only abnormality shown is a low K_{CO}.

2. A classic cause of reduced K_{CO} with normal spirometry is anaemia. This patient should have a full blood picture analysed as a first-line measure.

Case 92

A 36-year-old woman has been attending the respiratory outpatient department for 5 years because of sarcoidosis. Her disease has been well controlled recently, and her dose of oral steroids has been gradually reduced over a period of several months. On her most recent visit, she complains of increasing shortness of breath over the preceding 3 weeks. Her pulmonary function tests are shown alongside a set taken when she was feeling well.

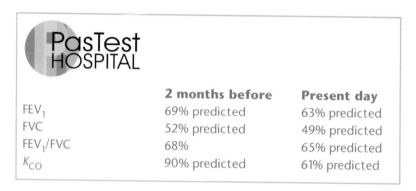

PasTest HOSPITAL

	2 months before	Present day
FEV$_1$	69% predicted	63% predicted
FVC	52% predicted	49% predicted
FEV$_1$/FVC	68%	65% predicted
K_{CO}	90% predicted	61% predicted

What parameter has changed significantly between the two sets of readings, and how would you account for this?

Answer 92

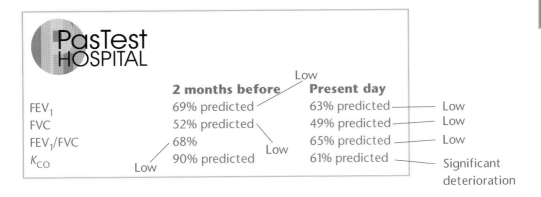

PasTest
HOSPITAL

	2 months before	Low **Present day**	
FEV₁	69% predicted	63% predicted	Low
FVC	52% predicted	49% predicted	Low
FEV₁/FVC	68%	65% predicted	Low
K_CO	Low 90% predicted Low	61% predicted	Significant deterioration

The FEV$_1$ and FVC remain fairly similar between both sets of readings, indicating a restrictive lung defect. The major deterioration lies with the K_{CO}, which has taken a marked turn for the worse. This is most likely due to a deterioration in the underlying disease process because of the reducing dose of steroids. Consideration should be given to increasing the steroid dose.

INTERPRETING BEDSIDE CHART DATA

14

INTERPRETING BEDSIDE CHART DATA

The most basic and readily available data on a patient lie at the end of the bed. Nursing staff dutifully complete a number of observations on a regular basis. The nature of these and the frequency at which they are taken vary depending on the clinical status of the patient. The basic observations on all patients include: heart rate, blood pressure, temperature, respiratory rate and blood oxygen saturation (SpO_2) (see box below). These are often termed the 'vital signs'. Specialist units (such as neurosurgery) and intensive care units (ICUs)/high dependency units (HDUs) have the most detailed range of recordings reflecting the severity of illness.

DON'T FORGET
The best way to learn from bedside charts is to pick them up on the ward during clinical attachments

Analysis and interpretation of bedside chart data are an extension to the clinical assessment of a patient. It may also provide the first evidence of a downward trend in the clinical condition, potentially allowing one to act before the deterioration is irreversible.

DON'T FORGET
Data interpretation begins at the end of the bed

Also found at the end of the bed are a fluid balance chart and drug chart – these are equally valuable sources of information.

BASIC OBSERVATIONS MEASURED (WITH NORMAL RANGES)

Pulse rate	60–100 beats per minute
Blood pressure	90/60 mmHg to 135/85 mmHg
	(always compare current with baseline)
Respiratory rate	14–18 breaths per minute
Oxygen saturations	96–100% on room air
Temperature	36.5–37.5°C

There are also a number of charts used for specific indications. An example of this is the stool chart (see page 344). For those with altered bowel habit this offers the doctor an insight into the patient's motions over a 24-h period. The frequency and consistency of the stools along with the presence of blood or mucus are recorded.

The pattern of observations is as important as a single snapshot of observations, as shown by the example below in a patient with a swinging fever.

Fig 14.1: Swinging fever

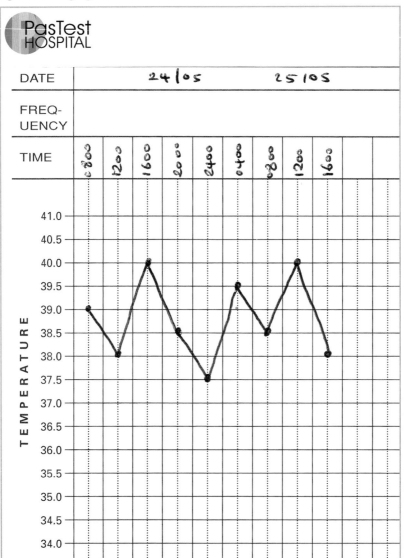

The process of placing a patient on specialist observation charts is based on clinical suspicion that the patient may come to harm unless changes are noted swiftly and acted upon. Perhaps one of the cases most illustrative of this point is a patient with a head injury being placed on a neurological observation chart.

The example below shows a neurological observation chart that documents the components of the Glasgow Coma Scale (GCS) at various points in time. At 11:00 hours the GCS drops from 14/15 to 7/15 and urgent action should be taken.

Fig 14.2: Sudden drop in GCS

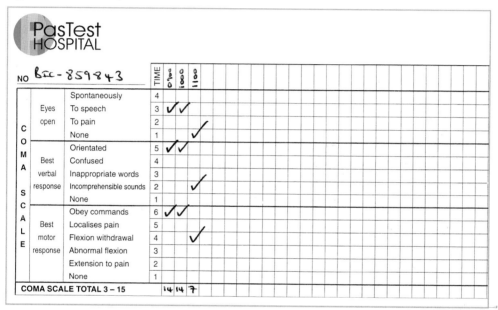

Drug charts

A great deal of information about a patient is found by looking at a drug chart. Not infrequently errors occur. Every doctor looking after an individual patient's care may prescribe medications and for this reason conflicting prescriptions may occur with potentially devastating consequences.

Case 93

FAECES CHART

NAME	A PATIENT	HOSPITAL NUMBER		123456
DATE OF BIRTH	1 / 1 /1970	WARD	ButterCup	

DATE	TIME	AMOUNT	CONSISTENCY	BLOOD	MUCUS	PUS	SIGN
10 /06	0800	MODERATE	LIQUID	✓	✓		
	1000	"	"	✓			
	1230	"	"	✓			
	1425	"	"		✓		
	1615	"	"	✓			
	1845	"	"	✓			
	2105	LARGE	"	✓	✓		
	2330	"	"	✓			
11/06	0200	"	"	✓	✓		
	0530	MODERATE	"	✓			
	0720	"	"	✓			
	0930	"	"	✓	✓		
	1145	"	"	✓	✓		
	1355	LARGE	"	✓	✓		
	1605	MODERATE	"	✓			
	1830	"	"	✓			
	2010	"	"	✓			
	2235	"	"	✓			
	2355	"	"	✓			

Summarise the findings on the stool chart and list the potential causes

Answer 93

This patient is having bowel motion activity recorded formally using a faeces chart. At least eight motions each day have been passed. The consistency has been liquid on all occasions. Furthermore it is mucoid and bloody. It would be important clinically for the fluid balance sheet to be assessed in conjunction with the stool chart to assess for adequate hydration. Possible causes for this pattern of bowel activity are listed in the box below.

Inflammatory bowel disease
Infective diarrhoea (eg *Shigella, Salmonella*)
Colorectal malignancy
Ischaemic colitis

Case 94

DAILY WEIGHTS		PasTest HOSPITAL
DATE	TIME	WEIGHT
10/06/05	0800 HRS	125 kc
11/06/05	0800	124 kc
12/06/05	0800	123.1 kc
13/06/05	0800	122.2 kc
14/06/05	0800	115.4 kc
15/06/05	0800	115.9 kc
16/06/05	0800	116.6 kc
17/06/05	0800	118.1 kc

1. **Explain the findings on this daily weight chart.**

2. **What could be the reason for the sudden loss of nearly 7 kg on 14/06/05?**

Answer 94

DAILY WEIGHTS		PasTest HOSPITAL
DATE	TIME	WEIGHT
10/06/05	0800 HRS	125 kg
11/06/05	0800	124 kg
12/06/05	0800	123.1 kg
13/06/05	0800	122.2 kg — Steady weight loss until here
14/06/05	0800	115.4 kg — dramatic weight loss
15/06/05	0800	115.9 kg
16/06/05	0800	116.6 kg
17/06/05	0800	118.1 kg — gradual weight gain

1. Daily weight charts are an extension of the standard fluid balance ('input/output') chart. In the short term (hours and days) changes usually reflect a change in body fluid content. It is paramount (as seen from the chart) that the recordings are taken at the same time each day. Dieticians keep weight records for those who are undernourished, receiving enteral or parenteral nutritional supplementation or enrolled in dietary programmes. In such cases, changes in the longer term become more important. The common reasons for recording daily weight are conditions in which excess fluid is retained by the body – severe congestive cardiac failure, ascites or nephrotic syndrome being prime examples.
   A response to treatment, in particular diuretics, and dietary sodium restriction may be monitored using a weight chart in conjunction with a fluid balance chart.
   This example documents a patient with significant ascites (excess fluid in the peritoneal cavity) over a period of several days following treatment. Over the initial 4 days a steady, albeit relatively small, daily reduction in weight is observed. This is in response to the introduction or increased dosing of diuretic therapy.

2. On 14/06/05 a more substantial reduction of 6.8 kg is observed. This is due to paracentesis with the removal of a substantial volume of fluid.

Case 95

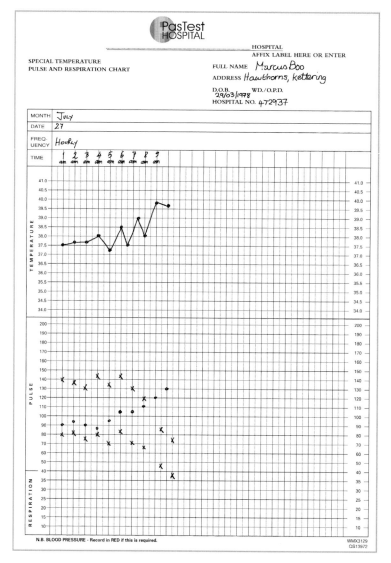

1. **Describe each abnormality on the observation chart and the overall impression.**

2. **Where should this patient be cared for?**

Answer 95

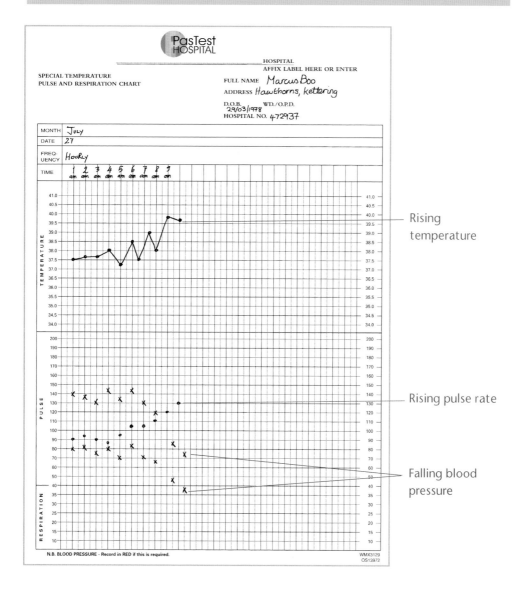

Rising temperature

Rising pulse rate

Falling blood pressure

1. The diagnosis of sepsis requires a full patient assessment. However, the bedside chart may provide the first evidence of impending sepsis. Taking an assessment of the chart over several hours, rather than a snapshot, aids in the diagnosis as one views the alteration of three key parameters – blood pressure, pulse rate and temperature. A persistent pyrexia or swinging fever is seen in the context of haemodynamic instability (hypotension and tachycardia).

   This example clearly shows a rising and sustained pyrexia with a maximum temperature of 39.9°C. A falling blood pressure, to a low of 78/38 mmHg, with an accompanying tachycardia of 130 beats/min demonstrates a haemodynamically unstable state.

2. If this patient fails to respond to initial treatment with fluids and antibiotics they should be transferred to an HDU/ICU environment where inotropic support (eg noradrenaline) may be administered to support the cardiovascular system until the underlying infection has been identified and treated.

Case 96

PasTest
HOSPITAL

.... HOSPITAL

AFFIX LABEL HERE OR ENTER

SPECIAL TEMPERATURE
PULSE AND RESPIRATION CHART

FULL NAME *Paul Bell*

ADDRESS *1 The Crescent, Bishop Stepford*

D.O.B. 22/01/79 WD./O.P.D. 5

HOSPITAL NO. *BIC 02 – 1234*

MONTH	
DATE	
FREQ-UENCY	
TIME	

| SpO₂ | 97% RA | 99% RA | 97% RA | 98% RA | 99% RA | 96% CA | 98% RA | 91% RA | 86% RA | 84% RA | 89% RA | 99% RA |

TEMPERATURE

41.0
40.5
40.0
39.5
39.0
38.5
38.0
37.5
37.0

Give your impression of the problem in this patient.

Answer 96

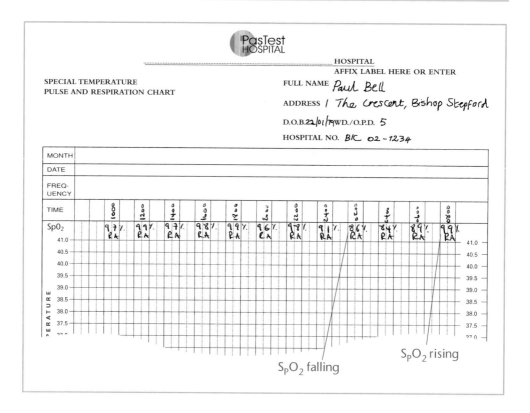

This chart outlines the blood oxygen saturations taken at 2-h intervals by pulse oximetry throughout a 24-h period. The vast majority are normal while breathing room air. If one was not to record the saturations during sleeping hours the patient may be deemed to be entirely normal. However, during the period 02:00–06:00 hours there is evidence of significant deoxygenation with a low of 84% at 04:00 hours.

The likely diagnosis here is obstructive sleep apnoea (OSA). If one was to waken the patient purposefully and then record the oxygen saturations they would probably return to normal. This diagnosis may be confirmed through formal sleep studies.

Case 97

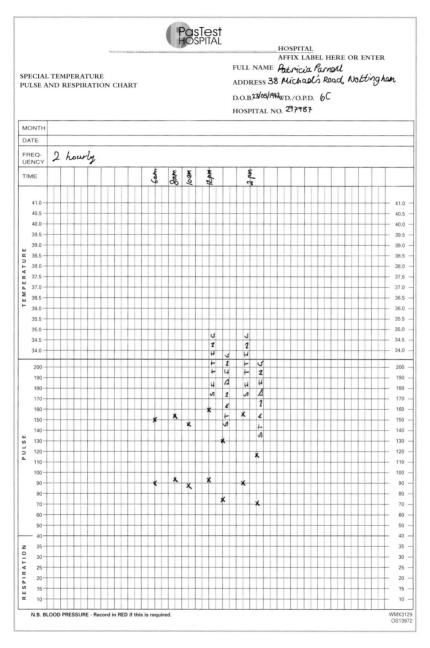

1. **What abnormality is seen?**

2. **Suggest a list of potential underlying diagnoses.**

Answer 97

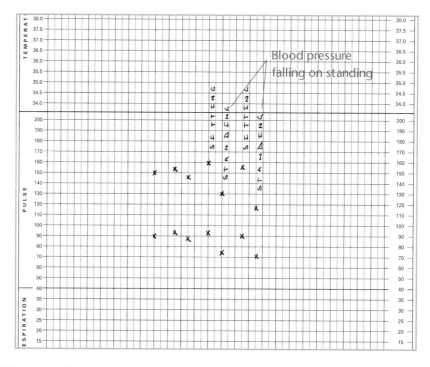

1. This basic chart demonstrates a series of blood pressure measurements. Unlike a conventional recording it indicates that some have been taken in different positions of posture. The likely indication for this is a patient with a history of falls, especially an elderly patient. For changes to be deemed significant, there must be a change in systolic blood pressure of greater than 20 mmHg when the patient changes from lying to standing. This patient has postural (orthostatic) hypotension.

2. Potential diagnoses are listed below:

CAUSES OF POSTURAL HYPOTENSION

Idiopathic
Dehydration (hypovolaemia)
Drug induced (eg diuretics, vasodilators, anti-parkinsonian medication)
Addison's disease (mineralocorticoid deficiency)
Autonomic neuropathy due to diabetes
Multi-system atrophy

Case 98

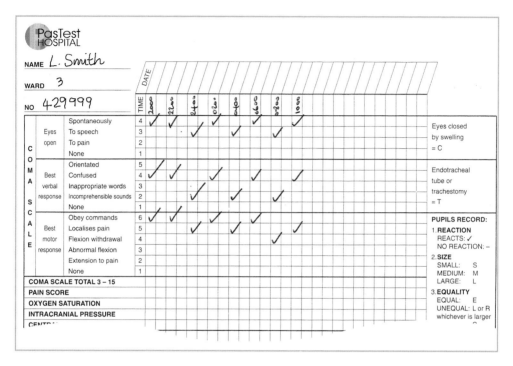

1. **Explain the findings on the neuro-observation chart.**

2. **What are the potential causes?**

Answer 98

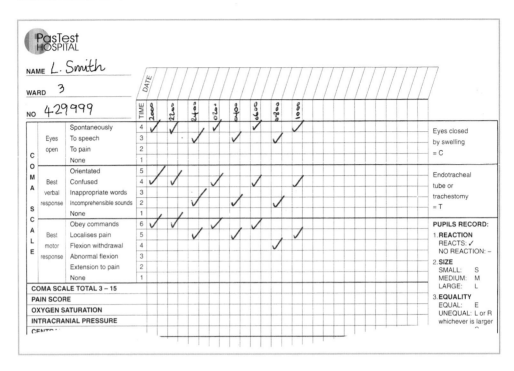

1. The GCS is a routinely used method of accurately and objectively recording a patient's level of consciousness. It is an easy to use scoring system which may be recorded in a reproducible fashion by nursing or medical staff. It comprises three independent categories – EYE OPENING, VERBAL RESPONSE and MOTOR RESPONSE. It is scored out of 15. The GCS must be measured in patients with head injury and after any neurosurgical intervention. This bedside chart illustrates its use in a patient following a fall.

    On admission the GCS is 14/15 on the basis of the patient being confused. At midnight the conscious level takes a drop from 14/15 to 10/15. Two hours later one can observe that the GCS has returned to its admission level of 14/15. Further frequent monitoring throughout the morning shows a repeat of this pattern – the GCS IS FLUCTUANT. An intracranial cause should be sought with urgent imaging.

2. This pattern is typically seen in subdural haematoma. Following a fall, the patient is lucid at times but the conscious level is variable. Extracranial causes, for example sepsis or hypoglycaemia, may also account for such patterns.

Case 99

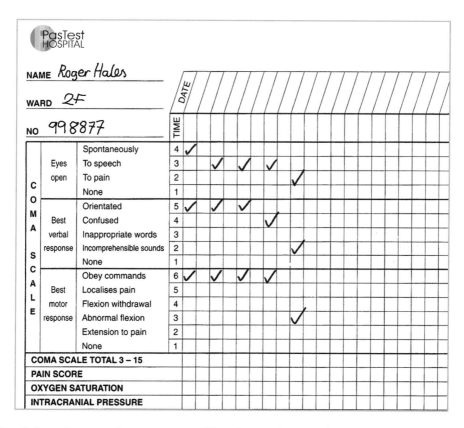

			TIME	4 ✓																	

PasTest HOSPITAL

NAME *Roger Hales*

WARD *2F*

NO *998877*

C O M A S C A L E	Eyes open	Spontaneously	4	✓																	
		To speech	3		✓	✓	✓														
		To pain	2					✓													
		None	1																		
	Best verbal response	Orientated	5	✓	✓	✓															
		Confused	4				✓														
		Inappropriate words	3																		
		Incomprehensible sounds	2					✓													
		None	1																		
	Best motor response	Obey commands	6	✓	✓	✓	✓														
		Localises pain	5																		
		Flexion withdrawal	4						✓												
		Abnormal flexion	3						✓												
		Extension to pain	2																		
		None	1																		
COMA SCALE TOTAL 3 – 15																					
PAIN SCORE																					
OXYGEN SATURATION																					
INTRACRANIAL PRESSURE																					

Explain what action one would take on becoming aware of these observations.

Answer 99

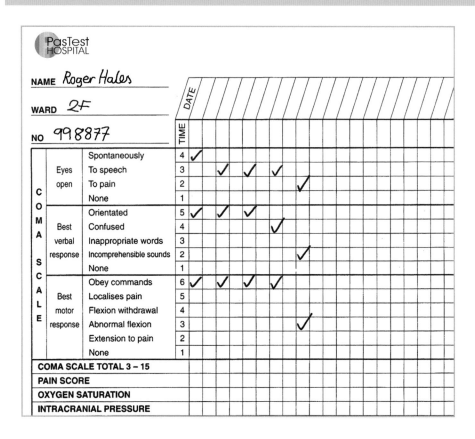

Changes in conscious level may be sudden and permanent as well as fluctuant. A significant drop in the GCS should be acted upon without delay. This bedside chart records a large drop from 13 to 7. This sudden change requires both a fast answer to establish the cause, and action to be taken to ensure the welfare of the patient. A GCS of less than 8/15 is an indication for consideration of intubation as the patient's airway is likely to become compromised .

CAUSES OF LARGE SUDDEN DROP IN GCS	
Intracerebral bleed (including subarachnoid haemorrhage)	Trauma – diffuse axonal injury
Cerebral oedema	Metabolic causes
Drugs and alcohol	(such as hypoglycaemia)

Case 100

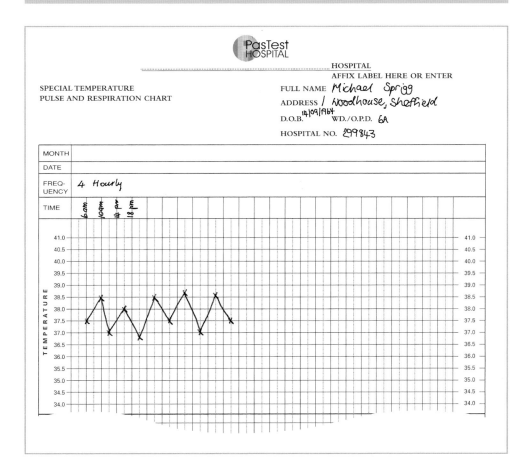

PasTest
HOSPITAL

.... HOSPITAL

AFFIX LABEL HERE OR ENTER

SPECIAL TEMPERATURE
PULSE AND RESPIRATION CHART

FULL NAME Michael Sprigg
ADDRESS 1 Woodhouse, Sheffield
D.O.B. 14/09/1964 WD./O.P.D. 6A
HOSPITAL NO. 299843

MONTH	
DATE	
FREQ-UENCY	4 Hourly
TIME	6am 10am 4 pm 18 pm

Describe the findings on this chart.

Answer 100

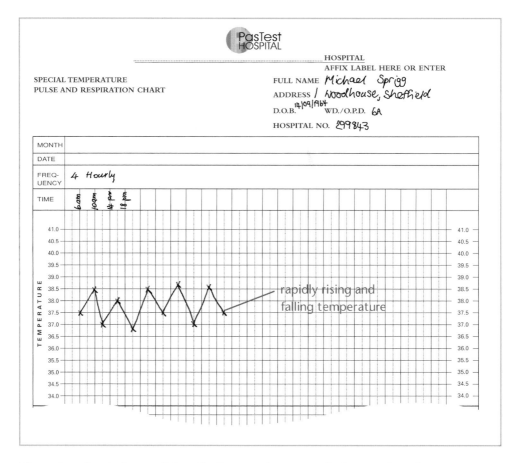

There is a simple but striking finding on the general observation chart over a period of several hours. The trend in temperature recordings is highly abnormal. It can be seen that the patient is apyrexic at times but has a significantly elevated temperature on other occasions. This is a swinging or spiking fever. Each temperature peak likely represents the shedding of bacterial toxins into the bloodstream. This finding may be due to any underlying infective source – although the pattern is characteristically seen in the setting of an abscess.

Case 101

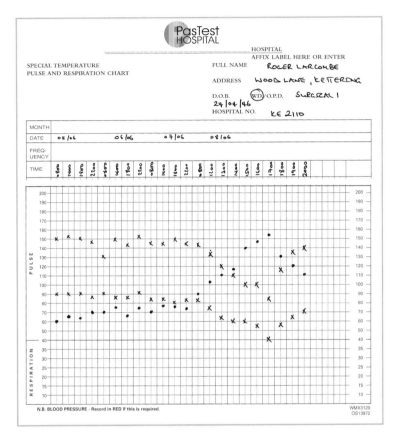

Describe the findings on these charts and what investigation(s) are needed to confirm the cause.

Answer 101

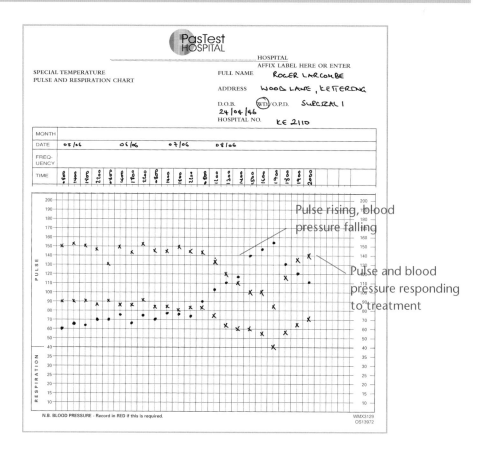

Most patients will have several observation charts at the end of the bed. These should all be viewed in a systematic fashion to maximise the information obtained. In this scenario, both the vital signs chart and the bowel habit chart reveal the likely diagnosis.

An inpatient for several days following admission with dark stools and rectal bleeding, this patient has remained stable, albeit with persistently abnormal bowel motions. It can be seen that on occasion the motion is both loose and dark in nature, but is always relatively small in volume and the patient's general observations initially remain normal.

Fluid resuscitation, possibly with blood products, has occurred. Note on day 4 (08/06) that the patient becomes progressively more tachycardic and with this the blood pressure falls. This corresponds to an increase in the frequency of the motions, which are noted to be black and foul smelling in nature – this patient has melaena.

The melaena has been present to an extent since admission, however, on this occasion the patient has become haemodynamically unstable. There has been a significant upper gastrointestinal tract bleed. The patient should now undergo emergency endoscopy to locate and if possible treat the cause. In the meantime, intravenous fluids and packed cells should be administered. Any coagulopathy should be corrected. One can see the blood pressure and tachycardia respond to fluid replacement (08/06 from 18:00 hours onwards).

Case 102

What electrolyte is likely to be deranged in this patient?

Answer 102

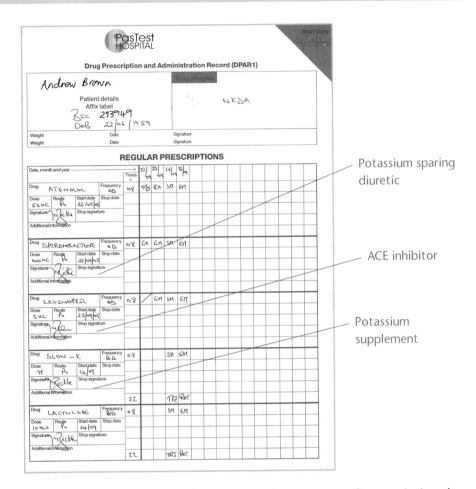

Potassium sparing diuretic

ACE inhibitor

Potassium supplement

This relatively simple drug chart illustrates the importance of appreciating the physiological actions of common medications and the problems that can arise. On admission, the patient is on a K⁺-sparing diuretic (spironolactone) at a dose that suggests an indication for liver disease rather than heart failure. On day 1 of his admission, an ACE inhibitor is introduced. The combination of an ACE inhibitor (lisinopril) and spironolactone, although acceptable, should be appreciated and initially the serum potassium should be checked to ensure it does not rise to a dangerous level. Therefore, when supplemental potassium is started the following day – perhaps by a busy doctor who does not usually cover this patient and who has limited understanding of the patient's overall case – we have a potential disaster. If left unchecked the K⁺ may increase to a level causing cardiac dysrhythmias or, worse, cardiac arrest.

Case 103

PasTest HOSPITAL

Start date
19/02/-5

Drug Prescription and Administration Record (DPAR1)

Drug allergies:

Patient details
Affix label

ASPIRIN

| Weight | Date | Signature | |
| Weight | Date | Signature | |

For the safety of the patient, please read the following instructions:
- Use generic names;
- Do not alter existing instructions;
- Discontinue a drug by drawing a line through it and signing.
- All drugs given must be initialled in the appropriate box.
- Write in CAPITALS and BLACK ink;
- Changes must be ordered by a new prescription;

REGULAR PRESCRIPTIONS

Date, month and year			Times

Drug CLOPIDOGREL	Frequency OD	08
Dose 75 MG	Route Po	Start date 19/02	Stop date
Signature	Stop signature
Additional information

Drug AMLODIPINE	Frequency OD	08
Dose 10 MG	Route Po	Start date 19/02	Stop date
Signature	Stop signature
Additional information

Drug WARFARIN	Frequency
Dose	Route	Start date	Stop date
Signature	Stop signature
Additional information SEE INR CHART

Drug PARACETAMOL	Frequency QDS	08
Dose 1G	Route Po	Start date 19/02	Stop date 21/02	12
Signature	Stop signature	16
Additional information		22

Drug ERYTHROMYCIN	Frequency QDS	08
Dose 250MG	Route Po	Start date 19/02	Stop date	12
Signature	Stop signature	16
Additional information		22

WMX 2139 011648

What has caused the difficulties in the INR level?

PasTest
HOSPITAL

Date	INR result	Warfarin dose	Prescribed by	Given by	Time	Date	INR result	Warfarin dose	Prescribed by	Given by	Time
19/02	2·35	4 MG	7G8	GM	2200						
20/02	/	4 MG	7G8	GM	2200						
21/02	2·98	3 MG	PKH	EFF	2200						
22/02	/	3 MG	7G8	KRT	2200						
23/02	3·99	2 MG	PKH	NHY	2200						

Answer 103

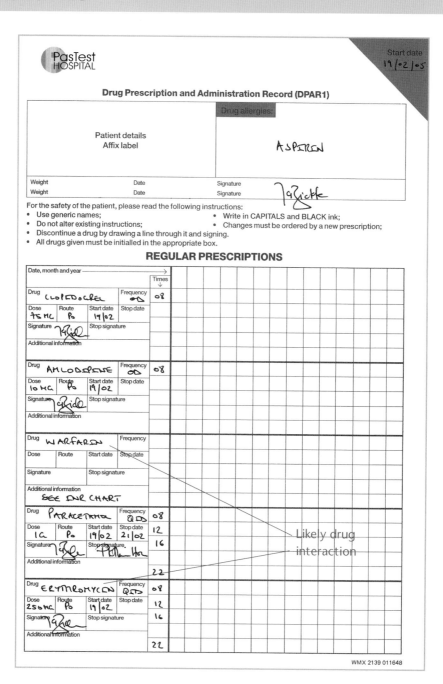

PasTest HOSPITAL

Date	INR result	Warfarin dose	Prescribed by	Given by	Time	Date	INR result	Warfarin dose	Prescribed by	Given by	Time
19/02	2·35	4 mg	7a8	CM	2200						
20/02	/	4 mg	7a8	CM	2200						
21/02	2·98	3 mg	PKH	EFF	2200						
22/02	/	3 mg	7a8	KRT	2200						
23/02	3·99	2 mg	PKH	NHY	2200						
			Rising INR								

April 2004

This scenario is based upon both a patient's drug chart and warfarin chart. Those patients on warfarin whilst in hospital should be placed on a dedicated warfarin chart. This generally outlines the indication for its prescription, the desired target INR (international normalised ratio) range and the daily warfarin dose and INR if taken. It is easy, but also dangerous, to view this chart in isolation. Following this patient's admission they are started on erythromycin and the warfarin dose remains at their usual level from admission. The INR was recorded before the first inpatient dose and was 2.35, perfectly placed in the desired range for the indication, atrial fibrillation. On day 3 it is checked again and is found to be 2.98. The dose is decreased by 1 mg, but again 2 days later the INR has continued to rise to 3.99. This is not in the highly dangerous range, but is enough to warrant consideration. The drug erythromycin is the cause. A macrolide antibiotic, it is known to enhance the anticoagulant effect of warfarin through its effect as an enzyme inhibitor in the liver.

MISCELLANEOUS 15

MISCELLANEOUS

Ankle brachial pressure index

The ankle brachial pressure index (ABPI) is an easily measured clinical parameter that is often used to assess the adequacy of blood flow to the lower limbs.

The patient should lie flat on a bed when having an ABPI measured. The systolic blood pressure in the brachial artery is measured using a stethoscope and sphygmomanometer. The systolic blood pressure at the ankle is then measured using a sphygmomanometer wrapped around the calf and a Doppler probe positioned over the posterior tibial or dorsalis pedis artery. Cuff pressure is inflated until blood flow to the foot is cut off. Flow is slowly re-established by deflating the cuff, and the pressure at which the first Doppler signal is obtained is noted.

After performing these tests, the observer will have two figures – the systolic blood pressures in the brachial artery and at the ankle. The ABPI is calculated simply by finding their ratio. In health, the ratio should be greater than or equal to 1. As the value decreases, symptoms and signs of arterial insufficiency to the lower limbs would be expected. Values lower than 0.5 may result in critical ischaemia. ABPIs of lower than 0.2 can be associated with ulceration and gangrene.

ABPI	INTERPRETATION
>1	Normal
<0.5	At risk of critical ischaemia
<0.2	At risk of ulceration and gangrene

One potentially complicating factor relates to the fact that some patients (particularly those with long-standing diabetes mellitus) have calcified arteries which cannot be compressed with a blood pressure cuff. In such cases, Doppler signals will be obtained even when the cuff is inflated to very high pressures. ABPIs cannot be reliably measured in these patients.

> **DON'T FORGET**
> The ABPI must be interpreted with caution in patients with diabetes mellitus

Case 104

A 74-year-old woman attends the diabetes clinic for a routine appointment. Her medical history includes type 2 diabetes (diagnosed 15 years previously), two previous myocardial infarctions and previous varicose vein surgery. She has noticed an ulcer on her left leg. Examination reveals the presence of varicose eczema, and a 4-cm-diameter shallow ulcer affecting the medial aspect of the left leg.

1. **How would you manage this woman?**

The ABPI was 0.9.

2. **What treatment should the patient receive?**

Answer 104

1. Leg ulcers can be the result of several underlying disease processes. Most commonly, ulcers can be due to venous insufficiency, arterial insufficiency or a combination of both. The patient's medical history puts her at risk of both venous (previous varicose vein surgery) and arterial (diabetes and ischaemic heart disease) ulcers. Findings on examination are, however, more in keeping with a venous ulcer.
   Management of venous ulceration is complex, but the mainstay relies on graduated pressure bandages. However, these bandages can exacerbate arterial insufficiency, and should not be routinely applied to all patients without first performing an ABPI measurement. The first step in the management of this patient's ulcer should therefore involve measurement of the ABPI.

2. The patient should be treated with graduated pressure bandages. Patients with an ABPI of less than 0.8 should not, in general, have compression bandages applied.

Synovial fluid analysis

Patients with acute monoarthritis often have synovial fluid aspirated for diagnostic purposes. It is important to be able to differentiate between the common causes of the acutely red, hot and swollen joint on the basis of fluid analysis.

DIAGNOSIS	APPEARANCE	LEUKOCYTE COUNT (PER mm^3)	APPEARANCE ON PLANE POLARISED LIGHT MICROSCOPY
Septic arthritis	Purulent	>750,000	
Haemarthrosis	Heavily bloodstained		
Gout	Cloudy	3000–40,000	Negatively birefringent needle-shaped crystals
Pseudogout	Cloudy	3000–40,000	Weakly positively birefringent rhomboidal crystals

MEMORY AID

Gout – remember the letter 'N' – **N**egatively birefringent, **N**eedle-shaped crystals of sodium urate

Pseudogout – remember the letter 'P' – weakly **P**ositively birefringent rhomboidal crystals of sodium **P**yrophosphate

Schirmer's test

Keratoconjunctivitis sicca is the term used to describe dry eyes. This phenomenon can occur in isolation (primary Sjögren's syndrome) or in association with many other rheumatological conditions.

The test is performed by attaching a specially shaped piece of filter paper to the lower eyelid. This is left for 5 min, and the distance that has become wet is then measured. Normally 10 mm or more of the paper will become wet.

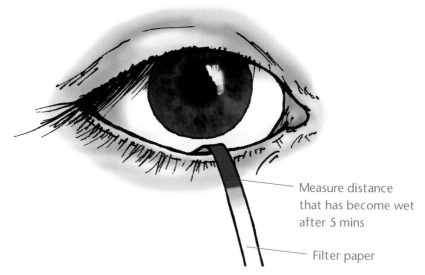

Measure distance
that has become wet
after 5 mins

Filter paper

Fig 15.1

It is important to bear in mind, however, that normal tear production is reduced in old age. Also, drugs with anticholinergic properties, such as tricyclic antidepressants, reduce tear production and may result in a false-positive Schirmer's test.

PABA test

The PABA test is used to detect pancreatic exocrine insufficiency, ie failure of the pancreas to produce sufficient enzymes for complete digestion.

The principle behind the test is simple. After fasting overnight, the patient is given a fixed dose of a peptide comprising *N*-benzoyl-L-tyrosyl-para-aminobenzoic acid (NBT-PABA). In a patient with normal pancreatic exocrine function, pancreatic enzymes break down NBT-PABA into the smaller compound PABA, which is then absorbed and excreted in the urine. Normally more than 70% of the dose administered appears in the urine. Less than 70% excretion implies that the exocrine activity of the pancreas is impaired.

DON'T FORGET

Normally >70% of the oral PABA dose is detected in the urine

Tests for the presence of *Helicobacter pylori*

The Gram-negative bacillus *H. pylori* can infect the stomach and predispose to the development of peptic ulcer disease. Testing for the presence of the organism should be carried out in all patients with a peptic ulcer, and eradication should be attempted in affected individuals.

There are several methods that can be used to test for the presence of *H. pylori*.

Breath testing

This test relies on the fact that *H. pylori* organisms produce urease, an enzyme that breaks down urea to form ammonia and carbon dioxide. The ammonia produced raises the pH and helps the organism survive the acidic environment in the stomach.

In a *H. pylori* breath test, the patient is given a tablet containing radiolabelled urea ([^{13}C]urea). If infection is present, the organisms act on the urea to liberate radiolabelled carbon dioxide ($^{13}CO_2$). A sample of breath is collected (eg in a tube or balloon), and analysed for the presence of $^{13}CO_2$. If this is detected, the test is positive and the patient can be assumed to be infected.

This test rapidly becomes negative if *H. pylori* is eradicated.

Detection of *H. pylori* antibodies

A sample of blood can be tested for the presence of IgG antibodies to *H. pylori*. The test can remain positive for up to a year after eradication therapy, and so it is not a particularly useful way of testing for clearance.

Campylobacter-like organism (CLO) test

This test also requires a biopsy sample obtained at OGD. The sample of tissue is placed into a medium that contains urea and phenol red. Phenol red is a dye that turns red in alkaline conditions. If *H. pylori* is present in the biopsy sample, its urease enzyme will liberate ammonia from the urea in the medium, causing the pH to rise. The colour of the medium will therefore turn red (Figure 2).

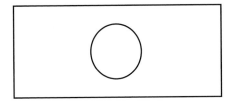

CLO test negative

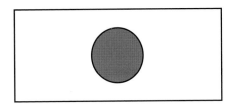

CLO test positive (red circle)

Fig 15.2

Tissue histology

A stomach biopsy sample can be stained and examined under a microscope. This may reveal curved organisms at the mucosal surface.

Tissue culture

A biopsy sample obtained at oesophago-gastro-duodenoscopy (OGD) can be cultured to look for the presence of offending organisms.

Audiograms

Audiograms illustrate, in graphical form, how well a person can hear noises at different frequencies. A healthy ear can hear sounds transmitted in the air better than those conducted by bone. This is because the ossicles in the middle ear amplify sound waves in the air.

Several patterns of abnormalities should be recognised.

1. **Conductive deafness**

   Anything that impedes the progression of sound waves down the ear canal can result in conductive deafness. The classical example of this is the patient with severe ear wax. In these conditions, sounds conducted by bone will be heard louder than those conducted by air. The audiogram will show a gap between the hearing level for air and bone conduction. This is termed a wide air–bone gap.

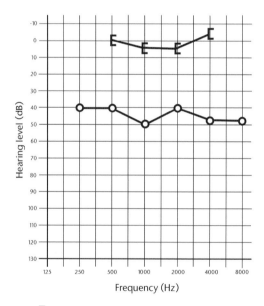

[Bone conduction (right ear)
O Air conduction (right ear)

Fig 15.3

2. **Sensorineural deafness**

A patient with unilateral auditory nerve damage (for example, due to an acoustic neuroma) will have reduced hearing for both air conduction and bone conduction.

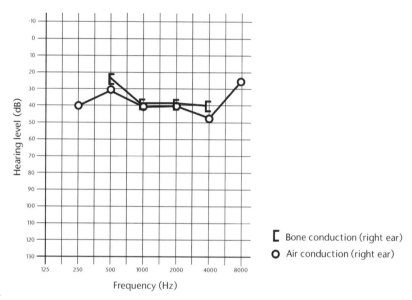

Fig 15.4

3. **Presbyacusis**

This describes the loss of hearing of sounds at high frequencies that is a common finding in elderly patients. It represents a form of sensorineural deafness.

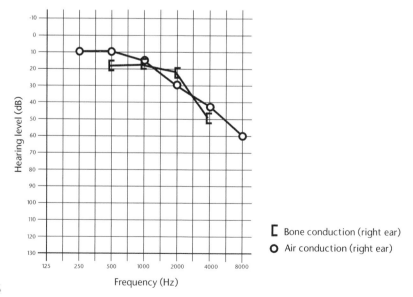

Fig 15.5

4. **Noise-induced hearing loss**

   Patients with noise-induced hearing loss typically have difficulty hearing sounds with a frequency around 4000 Hz. Their audiograms usually have a trough at this frequency level.

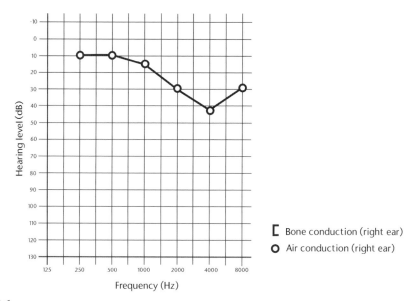

Fig 15.6

Cardiovascular risk

Until relatively recently, clinical judgement has been the main method of deciding which patients require drug therapy for primary prevention against cardiovascular disease. Guidelines are now available that aim to help doctors decide which patients require treatment. One part of a cardiovascular risk assessment chart is shown here.

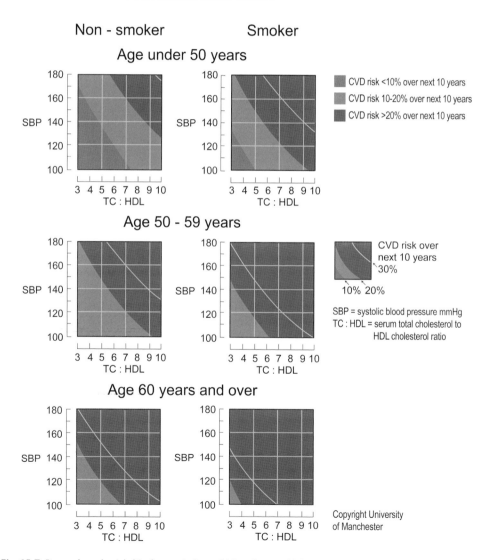

Fig 15.7 *Reproduced with kind permission of Manchester University Press*

These charts are easily interpreted as follows.

1. Choose the correct chart using the patient's sex, smoking status and age group. Whether or not a patient is classified as a smoker depends on their lifetime exposure to smoke, not just their current smoking status. Thus, patients who are ex-smokers, but gave up smoking within the last 5 years, should be classified as smokers for the purposes of interpreting these charts.

2. Knowledge of the patient's systolic blood pressure and details of their lipid profile are plotted to obtain the patient's cardiovascular risk over the next 10 years. Note that the x-axis on the charts plots the ratio of total cholesterol to high-density-lipoprotein (HDL) cholesterol, and this value should be used when available. When only the serum cholesterol concentration is known, assume that the HDL level is 1 mmol/l.

COMPLETE CLINICAL CASES

Use your understanding and interpretative skills from the rest of the book to approach these complete cases. The cases represent full patient pathways in which data from a multitude of investigations are available for interpretation. These holistic cases will test your skills in real life scenarios.

COMPLETE CLINICAL CASES

Case 105

DATA COVERED IN THIS CLINICAL CASE SCENARIO

- Toxicology blood levels
- Biochemistry: liver function tests
- Haematology: coagulation
- Imaging: chest X-ray
- Respiratory: arterial blood gas
- Microbiology: sputum
- Bedside chart: vital signs

An 18-year-old student is found by her housemates. She is in a confused state on the floor and is surrounded by several packets of paracetamol. It is 22:00 hours and they are able to ascertain that she took the tablets around 15:30 hours that day. She smells of alcohol. She had been on medications for low mood but is otherwise healthy. On arrival at hospital half an hour later blood tests were taken which are shown.

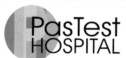

PasTest
HOSPITAL

Na^+	139 mmol/l
K^+	3.7 mmol/l
Urea	5.1 mmol/l
Creatinine	52 µmol/l
Cl^-	105 mmol/l
HCO_3^-	25 mmol/l
Paracetamol	160 mg/l
Alcohol	25 mmol/l
Salicylates	Nil
Bilirubin	12 µmol/l
AST	78 IU/l
ALT	65 IU/l
GGT	99 IU/l
ALP	67 U/l
Albumin	39 g/l
Prothrombin time	18.7 s
APTT	35.4 s
Fibrinogen	6.7 g/l

With the above results in mind outline the treatment approach for this patient.

Following the commencement of her treatment blood tests are taken on a regular basis and are shown below.

PasTest HOSPITAL

Time (hours)	Bilirubin (μmol/l)	AST (IU/l)	ALT (IU/l)	ALP (U/l)	GGT (IU/l)	Albumin (g/l)	PTT (s)
4	13	44	56	65	64	42	16.05
12	15	44	56	65	64	41	17.05
20	16	8001	7056	55	64	39	17.15
28	16	9977	10,230	75	54	38	18.55
36	19	12,333	11,156	65	61	34	19.05
44	23	12993	12,333	64	62	32	21.05
52	27	13,144	12,456	75	73	28	21.44
56	29	13,111	12,346	77	74	24	24.05
60	36	13,244	12,153	85	77	22	30.05

2. Outline the trend and significance of these results. What treatment should be considered now?

She is transferred to a regional centre where she undergoes surgery. In the initial days postoperatively she progresses well, but on day 5 becomes short of breath and a chest X-ray is taken which is shown below.

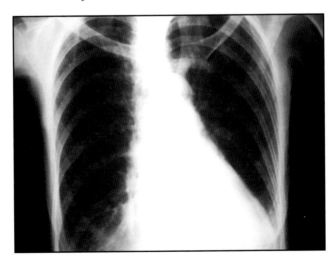

3. Report the findings on this chest X-ray.

At the same time a sample is sent for arterial blood gas analysis. The patient was breathing room air.

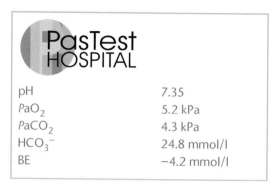

PasTest HOSPITAL	
pH	7.35
PaO_2	5.2 kPa
$PaCO_2$	4.3 kPa
HCO_3^-	24.8 mmol/l
BE	−4.2 mmol/l

4. What abnormality is observed on the arterial sample?

She is commenced on antimicrobial therapy and sputum is sent for analysis. The following day the results of her sputum analysis are conveyed from microbiology.

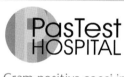

PasTest HOSPITAL

Gram-positive cocci in keeping with *Streptococcus pneumoniae*

During the middle of the night you are called by the nurse to see her as some of her vital signs are concerning. Her bedside chart is shown.

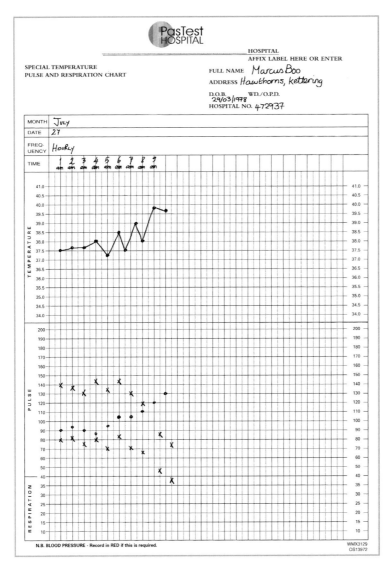

5. **Describe the findings on the chart and the underlying cause.**

Answer 105

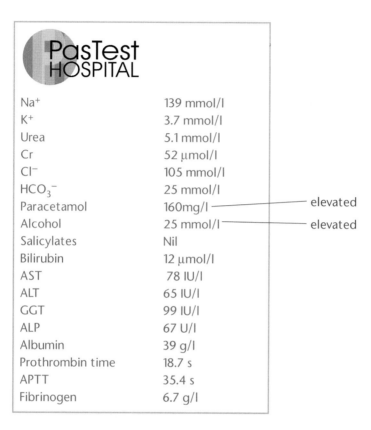

PasTest
HOSPITAL

Na$^+$	139 mmol/l
K$^+$	3.7 mmol/l
Urea	5.1 mmol/l
Cr	52 µmol/l
Cl$^-$	105 mmol/l
HCO$_3^-$	25 mmol/l
Paracetamol	160mg/l ——— elevated
Alcohol	25 mmol/l ——— elevated
Salicylates	Nil
Bilirubin	12 µmol/l
AST	78 IU/l
ALT	65 IU/l
GGT	99 IU/l
ALP	67 U/l
Albumin	39 g/l
Prothrombin time	18.7 s
APTT	35.4 s
Fibrinogen	6.7 g/l

1. The following should have been interpreted from the data provided in this scenario.

This woman has probably taken a substantial overdose of paracetamol in combination with alcohol.

The level of 160 mg/l is 6½ hours following ingestion. The significance of this is seen below on the paracetamol nomogram. At 6½ hours, the line intersects the normal treatment line of the graph at 125 mg/l making treatment necessary at levels higher than this: 160 mg/l is well above this line.

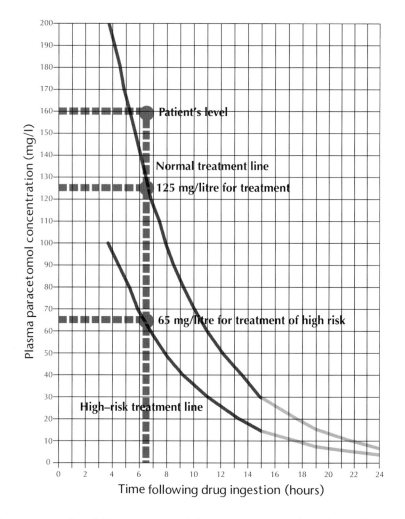

2. The patient should be treated with an intravenous infusion of *N*-acetylcysteine. The exact dose depends on the weight of the patient.

PasTest
HOSPITAL

Falling trend

Time (hours)	Bilirubin (μmol/l)	AST (U/l)	ALT (U/l)	ALP (U/l)	GGT (IU/l)	Albumin (g/l)	PTT (s)
4	13	44	56	65	64	42	16.05
12	15	44	56	65	64	41	17.05
20	16	8001	7056	55	64	39	17.15
28	16	9977	10,230	75	54	38	18.55
36	19	12,333	11,156	65	61	34	19.05
44	23	12993	12,333	64	62	32	21.05
52	27	13,144	12,456	75	73	28	21.44
56	29	13,111	12,346	77	74	24	24.05
60	36	13,244	12,153	85	77	22	30.05

Rising trend

This chart shows the changes in liver function over the 2–3 days following overdose. A huge surge in transaminases is seen from 20 hours indicating substantial hepatocelullar damage from the toxic effects of paracetamol. Hepatic necrosis is taking place and the liver is failing. This can be seen because the prothrombin time is rising and the albumin is falling, as the ability of the liver to synthesise protein is diminishing. A liver transplant should be considered.

3. Her transfer to a regional centre was to facilitate liver transplantation. Five days following her operation her chest X-ray, sputum analysis and ABG indicate that she had developed a postoperative pneumonia.

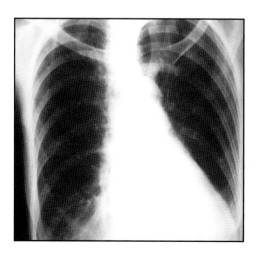

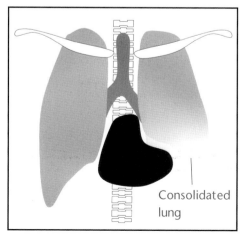

Consolidated lung

CXR REPORT

This is a PA chest radiograph taken on 14 December 2005. It is the second in a series of postoperative films on this patient. The patient is 18 years of age and is an inpatient on the liver unit. The technical quality of the film is sound. The most obvious abnormality on this film is an area of increased radio-opacity at the left base of the lung. There is loss of the left hemi-diaphragm silhouette. These findings are in keeping with consolidation. On review of the remainder of the film no other abnormalities are noted. These findings are in keeping with a left basal pneumonia. I would like to view previous films for comparison.

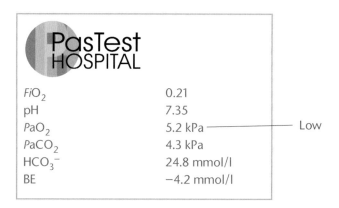

PasTest HOSPITAL		
FiO_2	0.21	
pH	7.35	
PaO_2	5.2 kPa	Low
$PaCO_2$	4.3 kPa	
HCO_3^-	24.8 mmol/l	
BE	−4.2 mmol/l	

4. The arterial blood gas shows a marked hypoxia with a normal pH.
   She has type 1 respiratory failure, caused by pneumonia.
   From the sputum analysis a specific causative organism has been identified
   – *Streptococcus pneumoniae*. It must be emphasised that culturing takes time.
   Treatment should be instigated with empirical therapy, and altered later, if
   necessary, on the basis of the growth and sensitivities.

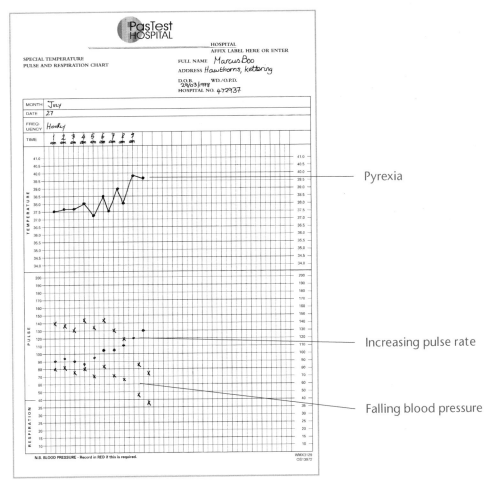

5. The bedside chart shows three key findings:

   1. Pyrexia

   2. Hypotension

   3. Tachycardia.

   In the context of an established pneumonia this may be in keeping with septic shock.

CASE SUMMARY

Paracetamol overdose requiring treatment
Development of hepatic failure requiring liver transplantation
Postoperative type 1 respiratory failure due to pneumonia
Development of septic shock

Case 106

DATA COVERED IN THIS CLINICAL CASE SCENARIO

- Bedside chart: neurological observations
- Imaging: CT brain
- Neurology: CSF analysis
- Neurology: EEG

A 38-year-old teacher is brought to hospital by her concerned husband due to her unusual behaviour and sleepiness over the past 48 h. She has recently returned from supervising a school trip.

Her observation chart from the initial 6 h of her admission is shown.

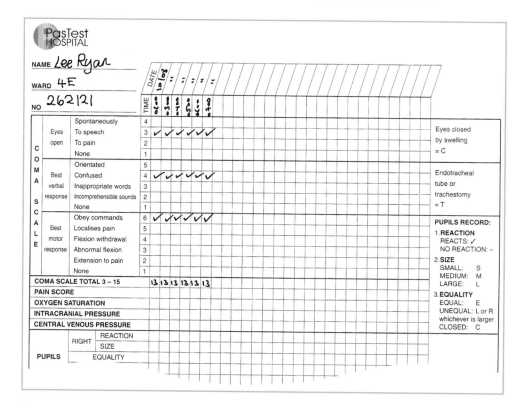

CT imaging of the brain is arranged and the following report is telephoned to her doctor.

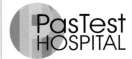

Neuroradiology Department
Routine un-enhanced images of the brain performed. No mass lesion seen. There is the suggestion of mild oedema within the temporal lobes bilaterally. MRI recommended.

Clinical examination revealed no signs of raised intracranial pressure. After discussion with the patient's consultant, lumbar puncture is performed. The details are below.

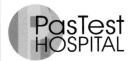

Opening pressure	16 mmH$_2$O
Appearance	Clear
	No organisms seen on microscopy
WCC	121 /mm^3 (>95% lymphocytes)
RCC	3 /mm^3
Glucose	2.8 mmol/l (plasma glucose 5.6 mmol/l)
Total protein	0.89 g/l (plasma total protein 0.44 g/l)

1. **Summarise the findings from the CSF analysis and suggest one further specific test that might be performed on the CSF given the clinical history.**

In the meantime an electroencephalogram is also performed. The report is sent back with the patient.

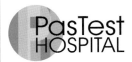

EEG Department
There is evidence of slow wave changes. Periodic complexes are seen

2. **Given the result of the EEG, CSF analysis and CT brain imaging what is the likely diagnosis?**

Answer 106

1. Given the finding of an altered conscious level, the patient is placed on a neuro-observation chart. The observation chart shows a stable Glasgow Coma Scale of 13/15. The patient is deemed to be confused and opens her eyes to speech.

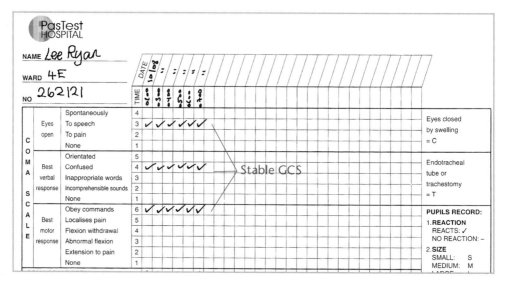

The CT brain imaging is abnormal. Lumbar puncture and an EEG are therefore performed to help come to a diagnosis.

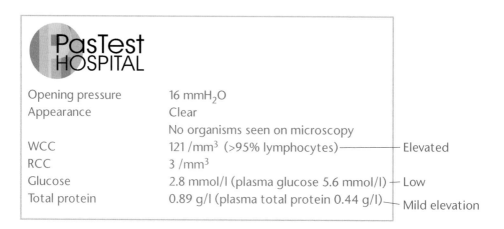

PasTest HOSPITAL		
Opening pressure	16 mmH$_2$O	
Appearance	Clear	
	No organisms seen on microscopy	
WCC	121 /mm^3 (>95% lymphocytes)	Elevated
RCC	3 /mm^3	
Glucose	2.8 mmol/l (plasma glucose 5.6 mmol/l)	Low
Total protein	0.89 g/l (plasma total protein 0.44 g/l)	Mild elevation

This collection of findings is termed a CSF pleocytosis.

CAUSES OF A CSF PLEOCYTOSIS

Viral meningitis
Encephalitis
Partially treated bacterial meningitis
TB or fungal meningitis
Intracranial abscess
Post-subarachnoid haemorrhage

One should have inferred from the clinical scenario so far that the cause of her symptoms and CSF findings is a viral meningitis/encephalitis. An additional test would be for PCR serology of the CSF to enable detection of viruses, especially herpes simplex virus (HSV).

2. The EEG findings demonstrate the characteristic neurophysiological findings of HSV encephalitis.
   Further tests in HSV encephalitis would include:

- **MRI of brain:**
  - Oedema within the temporal lobes bilaterally (better seen than on CT)
  - High signal within the temporal lobes
- **PCR serology of CSF**
  - HSV-1: present.

IN SUMMARY

A CSF pleocytosis
Herpes simplex encephalitis

Case 107

DATA COVERED IN THIS CLINICAL CASE SCENARIO

- Haematology: iron studies
- Biochemistry: liver function tests
- Genetics
- Peritoneal fluid analysis
- Haematology: coagulation

A 34 year-old oil-rig engineer is required to attend a medical before a secondment to his company's overseas operation in Brunei. He has been fortunate with his health with no previous attendance within the health service. He admits to smoking 20 cigarettes a day and drinking approximately 38 units of alcohol a week. His conscientious doctor sends several tests. The following results were of some concern.

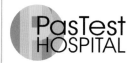

PasTest HOSPITAL	
Serum iron	99 µmol/l
Serum ferritin	878 µg/l
TIBC	12 µmol/l

1. **What can one infer from this iron profile?**

2. **Ferritin is an acute phase reactant. Name some other acute phase reactants.**

His liver function tests are recalled on the computer and are shown below.

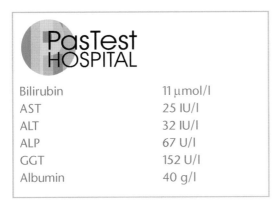

Bilirubin	11 µmol/l
AST	25 IU/l
ALT	32 IU/l
ALP	67 U/l
GGT	152 U/l
Albumin	40 g/l

3. What do the liver function tests show?

The doctor is concerned about an underlying genetic disorder and a blood sample is sent to the genetics laboratory. The result below was obtained.

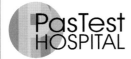

Genetics Laboratory

Homozygous abnormality on chromosome 6p – HFE gene – missense mutation C282Y

The doctor tries to arrange treatment, but unfortunately the patient leaves his job and no further medical action is taken. Nothing is heard of him for several years, until he is admitted to a local hospital with a distended abdomen and fever.

Physical examination demonstrates the presence of ascites. Peritoneal aspiration is performed and shown below.

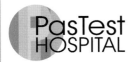

Neutrophil count (WCC)	312 cells/mm^3
Ascites albumin content	19 g/l
Serum albumin	32 g/l
Microscopy and Gram stain	Gram-negative rods
Culture	E. coli
Amylase	92 u/l

4. What is the diagnosis?

He is treated for the acute condition and further blood tests are performed to assess his liver function.

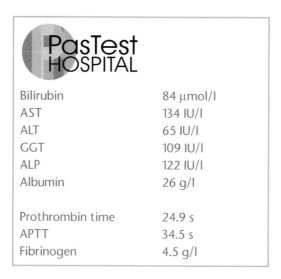

PasTest HOSPITAL	
Bilirubin	84 μmol/l
AST	134 IU/l
ALT	65 IU/l
GGT	109 IU/l
ALP	122 IU/l
Albumin	26 g/l
Prothrombin time	24.9 s
APTT	34.5 s
Fibrinogen	4.5 g/l

5. What do these liver function tests suggest?

Answer 107

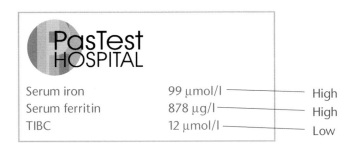

PasTest HOSPITAL		
Serum iron	99 µmol/l	High
Serum ferritin	878 µg/l	High
TIBC	12 µmol/l	Low

1. These results suggest a state of iron overload. The most likely reason for this in an otherwise healthy person found at screening is hereditary haemochromatosis. Haemochromatosis may present with:

   - Cardiomyopathy

   - Liver disease

   - Pituitary disease

   - Diabetes mellitus

   - Joint problems (pseudogout).

   All manifestations are related to the deposition of iron within organs.

2. Other acute phase reactants include:

   - CRP

   - ESR

   - Ceruloplasmin.

   Note that albumin acts as a 'negative acute phase reactant' – its levels decreasing with inflammation.

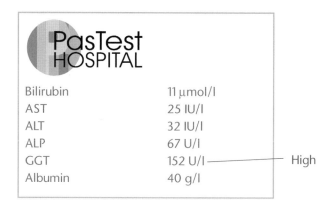

Bilirubin	11 μmol/l	
AST	25 IU/l	
ALT	32 IU/l	
ALP	67 U/l	
GGT	152 U/l	High
Albumin	40 g/l	

3. As is commonly the case, both at diagnosis and in established disease, the LFTs are essentially normal. The only abnormal LFT is the GGT which is mildly elevated. Given his clinical history this is likely to reflect heavy alcohol consumption rather than haemochromatosis.

Idiopathic haemochromatosis is an inherited autosomal recessive condition. Only homozygotes develop clinically overt disease. There is now a gene test for haemochromatosis and screening of first-degree relatives of patients is offered. The most common genetic defect is homozygosity of the C282Y missense mutation of the *HFE* gene on chromosome 6p. In addition, a different mutation – *H63D* – can play a role in some cases.

With appropriate management, patients with haemochromatosis should, in large part, not develop liver failure.

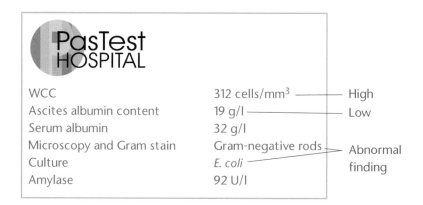

WCC	312 cells/mm^3	High
Ascites albumin content	19 g/l	Low
Serum albumin	32 g/l	
Microscopy and Gram stain	Gram-negative rods	Abnormal
Culture	E. coli	finding
Amylase	92 U/l	

4. The presentation with ascites implies the development of liver cirrhosis with portal hypertension. The peritoneal aspiration performed tells us three things:

   • The serum–ascites albumin gradient (SAAG) is 32 − 19 = 13 g/l. This tells us that the patient probably has portal hypertension.

- The ascitic fluid is infected with the Gram-negative rod *E. coli*.

- There is a high neutrophil count.

This all implies spontaneous bacterial peritonitis. In the acute setting, the most important result to note would be the WCC. An elevated WCC should be taken as evidence for peritonitis and appropriate therapy instituted before culture results are obtained. If the WCC had been normal, one should consider ascites secondary to the development of hepatocellular carcinoma. Haemochromatosis patients with cirrhosis are susceptible to this primary liver malignancy.

5. The accompanying LFTs show:

- Poor synthetic function (prothrombin time UP and albumin DOWN).

- Mildly deranged liver function.

- The patient has developed liver failure as a result of the combined hepatotoxic insults of iron and alcohol.

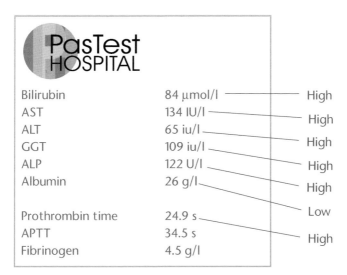

PasTest HOSPITAL		
Bilirubin	84 µmol/l	High
AST	134 IU/l	High
ALT	65 iu/l	High
GGT	109 iu/l	High
ALP	122 U/l	High
Albumin	26 g/l	Low
Prothrombin time	24.9 s	High
APTT	34.5 s	
Fibrinogen	4.5 g/l	

IN SUMMARY

Haemochromatosis
Spontaneous bacterial peritonitis
Liver failure

Case 108

- Haematology: full blood count
- Biochemistry: bone profile, urate and CRP
- Immunology: autoimmune screen
- Miscellaneous: knee aspirate analysis
- Respiratory: spirometry
- Imaging: chest X-ray and DEXA scan

A 39-year-old secretary attends hospital with a painful and swollen right knee, pains in the fingers and fatigue. The finger pains have been with her for several weeks and are especially bad first thing in the morning, making her work difficult. The knee is a more recent complaint.

On examination there is active synovitis in the small joints of the hands and a large effusion of the right knee.

Among the initial blood tests from the A&E officer are those shown.

PasTest
HOSPITAL

Hb	9.9 g/dl
MCV	89.9 fl
WCC	11.2 x 10^9/l
Platelets	199 x 10^9/l
Calcium	2.45 mmol/l
PO$_4^{3-}$	0.87 mmol/l
Albumin	36 g/l
Urate	0.34 mmol/l
CRP	312 mg/l

1. **Describe the findings.**

An enthusiastic junior doctor carries out knee aspiration, to exclude septic arthritis. The results are shown.

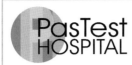

Specimen received	Synovial fluid from right knee
Appearance	Clear
Microscopy	< 2 leukocytes per mm^3
Plane polarised light microscopy	No crystals seen
Synovial fluid culture	No growth

A few days later the result of her autoimmune screen is sent to the ward.

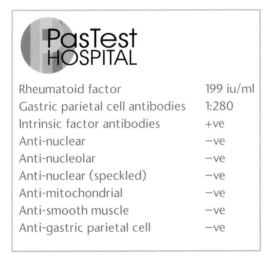

Rheumatoid factor	199 iu/ml
Gastric parietal cell antibodies	1:280
Intrinsic factor antibodies	+ve
Anti-nuclear	−ve
Anti-nucleolar	−ve
Anti-nuclear (speckled)	−ve
Anti-mitochondrial	−ve
Anti-smooth muscle	−ve
Anti-gastric parietal cell	−ve

She is treated for her arthritis and attends regular review for many years with a variable course to her illness. On one occasion she complains of increasing shortness of breath and on auscultation of the chest there are inspiratory crepitations at the bases.

Spirometry is arranged. The results are shown.

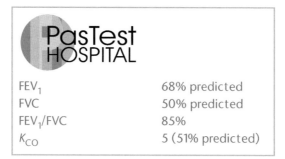

FEV$_1$	68% predicted
FVC	50% predicted
FEV$_1$/FVC	85%
K_{CO}	5 (51% predicted)

The accompanying chest X-ray is shown.

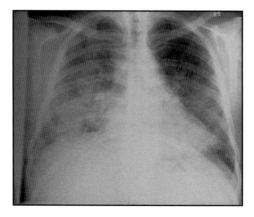

2. **What problem does this patient now have and how may it be related to her treatment?**

3. **What further radiological investigation would be of benefit?**

Six months later the patient sustains a forearm fracture. She is referred for a DEXA scan. The results can be seen below.

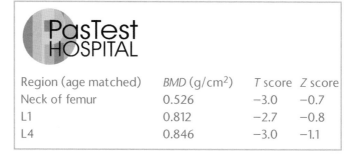

Region (age matched)	BMD (g/cm^2)	T score	Z score
Neck of femur	0.526	−3.0	−0.7
L1	0.812	−2.7	−0.8
L4	0.846	−3.0	−1.1

4. **Outline the significance of these results.**

Answer 108

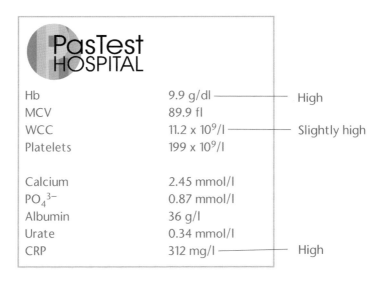

Hb	9.9 g/dl	High
MCV	89.9 fl	
WCC	11.2 x 10⁹/l	Slightly high
Platelets	199 x 10⁹/l	
Calcium	2.45 mmol/l	
PO₄³⁻	0.87 mmol/l	
Albumin	36 g/l	
Urate	0.34 mmol/l	
CRP	312 mg/l	High

1. The important findings from the FBC, bone profile and other biochemistry tests are:

   • A normocytic anaemia (low haemoglobin and normal MCV)

   • A substantially raised CRP

   • A normal urate

   • A normal bone profile.

   Sometimes normal blood results are as important as positive ones. In this case, gout is on the list of differential diagnoses for an acute-onset, painful, swollen joint so the urate level is important to measure. However, remember that the urate level can be normal in acute gout.

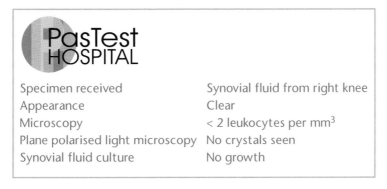

Specimen received	Synovial fluid from right knee
Appearance	Clear
Microscopy	< 2 leukocytes per mm³
Plane polarised light microscopy	No crystals seen
Synovial fluid culture	No growth

The knee aspirate sample is normal. No white cells or organisms were identified, and culture was negative, excluding septic arthritis. Similarly, no crystals were seen to suggest a crystalline arthritis.

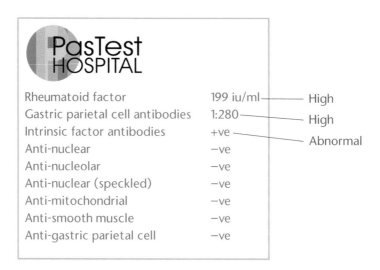

The result of the autoimmune screen is important. The rheumatoid factor is highly elevated, which in the context of the clinical symptoms and earlier finding of a raised CRP and normochromic anaemia imply a diagnosis of rheumatoid disease. There are three important points to remember about rheumatoid factor:

- Its level does not necessarily reflect disease activity

- It can be raised in a number of states other than rheumatoid disease (ie poor specificity)

- It does not need to be positive for the diagnosis of rheumatoid disease to be made (20% of patients are rheumatoid factor negative).

Interestingly, the screen has also antibodies to gastric parietal cells and intrinsic factor in keeping with a diagnosis of pernicious anaemia. It is common for patients to suffer from several coexisting autoimmune diseases.

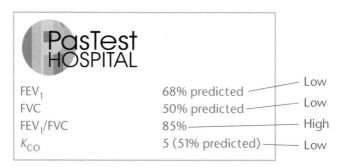

2. The positive findings from spirometry with transfer factor are:

- A reduced FEV_1

- A reduced FVC

- A high FEV_1/FVC ratio

- A reduced transfer factor.

This demonstrates a restrictive pattern wholly in keeping with interstitial lung fibrosis.

CHEST X-RAY REPORT

This is a PA chest X-ray of Mrs B taken on 2 January 2006. She is 39 years of age. The technical quality of the film is satisfactory. There is evidence of increased interstitial lung markings at both bases. The lung volumes appear reduced overall. These findings are typical of interstitial lung fibrosis. High-resolution computed tomography (HRCT) of the chest is advised.

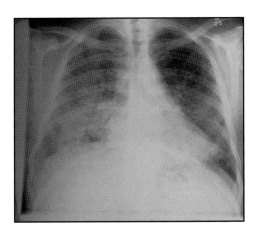 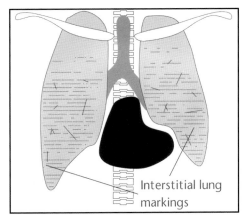

Interstitial lung markings

The presence of fibrosis may be due to:

- The disease itself – pulmonary fibrosis is one of the pulmonary manifestations of rheumatoid disease.

- A side effect of treatment with methotrexate (first-line disease-modifying anti-rheumatic drug treatment for this condition).

3. As seen in the report above HRCT is advisable as this will help clarify in greater detail the nature and extent of the disease.

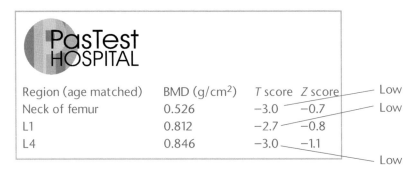

Region (age matched)	BMD (g/cm²)	T score	Z score	
				Low
Neck of femur	0.526	−3.0	−0.7	Low
L1	0.812	−2.7	−0.8	
L4	0.846	−3.0	−1.1	
				Low

4. Patients with rheumatoid disease often have exacerbations ('flares') of their disease requiring treatment with either intravenous or oral steroids. The disease itself and steroid treatment puts such patients at risk of developing osteoporosis which is diagnosed by dual energy X-ray absorptiometry (DEXA) scanning. A T score of less than −2.5 indicates osteoporosis. A score of −1.5 to −2.5 implies the presence of osteopenia.

IN SUMMARY

Knee effusion (due to rheumatoid disease)
Interstitial lung fibrosis (rheumatoid lung)
Steroid-induced osteoporosis

Case 109

DATA COVERED IN THIS CLINICAL CASE SCENARIO

- Respiratory: arterial blood gas
- Biochemistry: urea and electrolytes
- Bedside chart: fluid input/output
- Cardiology: ECG
- Imaging: abdominal X-ray

A 74-year-old man is admitted with a painful abdomen. He has a history of hypertension and atrial fibrillation. He had a laparotomy as a younger man for a gastric ulcer. He has not passed a motion in several days. On examination his abdomen is tender with rebound

An abdominal X-ray is taken and shown below.

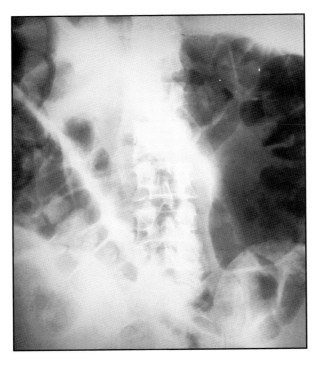

1. **Interpret this X-ray.**

The patient's condition rapidly deteriorates. An arterial blood gas is analysed.

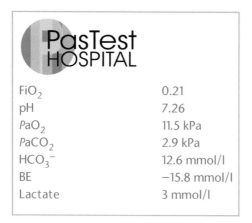

FiO_2	0.21
pH	7.26
PaO_2	11.5 kPa
$PaCO_2$	2.9 kPa
HCO_3^-	12.6 mmol/l
BE	−15.8 mmol/l
Lactate	3 mmol/l

2. Interpret this ABG.

The patient has emergency surgery. After a short stay in the high dependency unit (HDU) he returns to the ward. Several days later he complains of further abdominal discomfort after his patient-controlled analgesia (PCA) device is stopped. On examination he is tender in the suprapubic space and this area is dull to percussion. A urinary catheter has been *in situ* since surgery.

His fluid (input/output) chart is observed.

PasTest HOSPITAL

.... HOSPITAL.
AFFIX LABEL HERE OR ENTER
FULL NAME *John Dickens*
ADDRESS *2 Ford Street, Belfast*

DAILY FLUID CHART

D.O.B. *11a/04/1981* WD./O.P.D. *5*
HOSPITAL NO. *264567*

24 Hours
Beginning *26/01/2005*

TIME	INTAKE					OUTPUT					REMARKS
	BY MOUTH		INTRAVENOUS OR OTHER ROUTES			Urine ml.	Faeces ml.	Vomit ml.	Gast. Asp. ml.	Drain ml.	
	Amount ml.	Type	Amount ml.	Type	Add.						
0800			50			30					
0900			50			34					
1000			50			45					
1100			50			10					
1200			50			10					
1300			50			5					
1400			50			5					
1500			50			0					
1600			50			0					
1700			50			0					
1800			50			0					
1900											
2000											
2100											
2200											
2300											
2400											
0100											
0200											
0300											
0400											
0500											
0600											
0700											

DATE:-

INTAKE				Name				
TOTAL	By Mouth	Intravenous or Other Routes		Urine	Faeces	Vomit	Gast. Asp.	Drain
Day Total	ML	ML		ML	ML	ML	ML	ML
Night Total	ML	ML		ML	ML	ML	ML	ML
Total for 24 hours	ML	ML		ML	ML	ML	ML	ML

TOTAL INTAKE [   ]   TOTAL OUTPUT [   ]

WGA 225/04 10/200

3. **Describe the findings.**

Blood and urine are sent for analysis

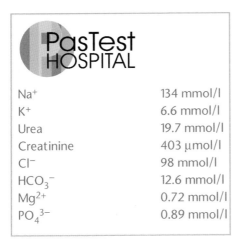

PasTest
HOSPITAL

Na^+	134 mmol/l
K^+	6.6 mmol/l
Urea	19.7 mmol/l
Creatinine	403 µmol/l
Cl^-	98 mmol/l
HCO_3^-	12.6 mmol/l
Mg^{2+}	0.72 mmol/l
PO_4^{3-}	0.89 mmol/l

4. **What problem has occurred?**

Immediate treatment is given for hyperkalaemia.

5. **An ECG was done just before treatment. Describe the findings on the ECG seen below.**

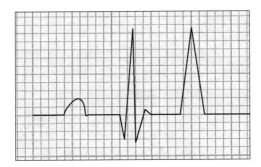

Answer 109

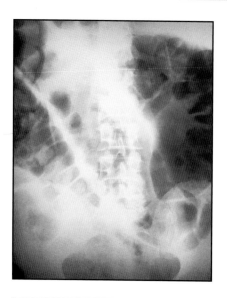 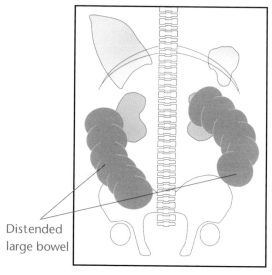

Distended
large bowel

 PasTest
HOSPITAL

Abdominal X-ray report

This is a supine AXR of Mr D taken on 13 January 2006. The patient is 74 years of age. The technical quality is adequate.

The distribution of gas within the large bowel is abnormal. The luminal diameter is 7 cm at the splenic flexure. Haustral markings can be seen. There is a paucity of gas beyond this point. No extraluminal gas is seen.

2. Interpretation of the ABG.

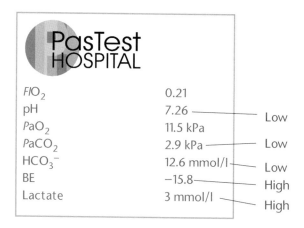

PasTest
HOSPITAL

FIO_2	0.21	
pH	7.26	Low
PaO_2	11.5 kPa	
$PaCO_2$	2.9 kPa	Low
HCO_3^-	12.6 mmol/l	Low
BE	−15.8	High
Lactate	3 mmol/l	High

The findings on arterial blood analysis are:

- Oxygenation is adequate.

- A low pH. This patient is profoundly acidotic.

- A low $PaCO_2$. Respiratory compensation is occurring.

- A low HCO_3^-. The origin of excess acid is metabolic in nature.

- A high lactate. This is a 'rogue' acid being produced in large quantities. In this case ischaemia of the large bowel is the cause.

The anion gap can be calculated:

$$\text{Anion Gap} = (Na^+ + K^+) - (Cl^- + HCO_3^-) = 23.6 \text{ mmol/l}$$

3. This patient has a high anion-gap metabolic acidosis, most likely due to lactic acidosis, secondary to an ischaemic bowel.

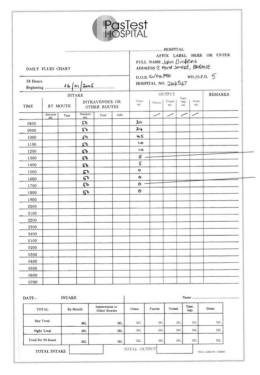

Poor urine output

Anuric

One should infer from the bedside chart that:

- there is a significant positive balance

- the urine output has tailed off in the last 4 hours.

- prior to becoming anuric the urine output was poor.

4. This patient has anuria which was preceded by a period of oliguria. In the first instance the urinary catheter should be checked and flushed to ensure there is no blockage.

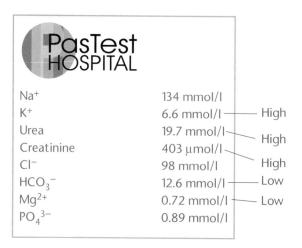

PasTest
HOSPITAL

Na^+	134 mmol/l	
K^+	6.6 mmol/l	High
Urea	19.7 mmol/l	High
Creatinine	403 μmol/l	
Cl^-	98 mmol/l	High
HCO_3^-	12.6 mmol/l	Low
Mg^{2+}	0.72 mmol/l	Low
PO_4^{3-}	0.89 mmol/l	

The blood results show that this patient has developed acute renal failure. From the clinical history it appears that this is due to obstruction of the renal tract.

The patient has life-threatening hyperkalaemia. A potassium of greater than 6.5 (in the context of acute renal failure) requires immediate treatment.

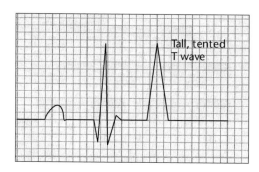

Tall, tented
T wave

5. The ECG shows classic changes related to hyperkalaemia. The T waves are tall and peaked.

IN SUMMARY

Large bowel obstruction
Bowel ischaemia with metabolic acidosis
Acute renal impairment (due to bladder obstruction)
ECG abnormality (due to hyperkalaemia)

Case 110

- Biochemistry: urea, electrolytes and CRP
- Haematology: full blood picture (FBP)
- Imaging: chest X-ray
- Respiratory: arterial blood gas
- Pleural fluid analysis
- Microbiology: stool analysis

A 54-year-old pilot is admitted to the local hospital with a complaint of increasing shortness of breath. He has noted this especially whilst flying recently and he has been seen by his occupational health doctor and prohibited from flying until investigation has been undertaken. He also complains of a cough and intermittent fever.

On examination the trachea is sited centrally. The left lung base is dull to percussion, vocal resonance is decreased and breath sounds are decreased.

Included in your initial investigations are a chest X-ray, FBP, U&E, CRP and ABG. All are shown below for interpretation.

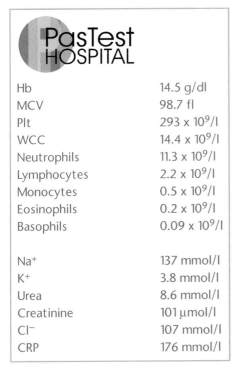

Hb	14.5 g/dl
MCV	98.7 fl
Plt	293 x 10^9/l
WCC	14.4 x 10^9/l
Neutrophils	11.3 x 10^9/l
Lymphocytes	2.2 x 10^9/l
Monocytes	0.5 x 10^9/l
Eosinophils	0.2 x 10^9/l
Basophils	0.09 x 10^9/l
Na$^+$	137 mmol/l
K$^+$	3.8 mmol/l
Urea	8.6 mmol/l
Creatinine	101 µmol/l
Cl$^-$	107 mmol/l
CRP	176 mmol/l

1. **What abnormalities are seen?**

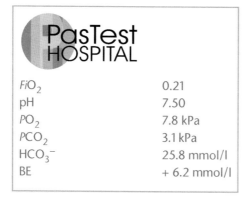

PasTest HOSPITAL	
FiO_2	0.21
pH	7.50
PO_2	7.8 kPa
PCO_2	3.1 kPa
HCO_3^-	25.8 mmol/l
BE	+ 6.2 mmol/l

2. Describe the findings on this ABG.

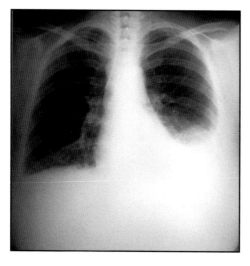

3. Comment on this chest X-ray.

A decision is made to perform a pleural tap for diagnostic purposes based on the findings from the initial investigations. The results are shown.

PasTest HOSPITAL	
Total protein	38 g/l
LDH	246 U/l
pH	7.37
Microscopy	Gram-negative rods

4. How would you interpret these results?

He is treated with a cephalosporin antibiotic based on known sensitivities. Three days into this treatment he develops diarrhoea. Stool samples are sent by his nurse. The result is shown below.

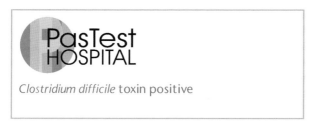

PasTest
HOSPITAL

Clostridium difficile toxin positive

5. What is the best course of action based on these findings?

Answer 110

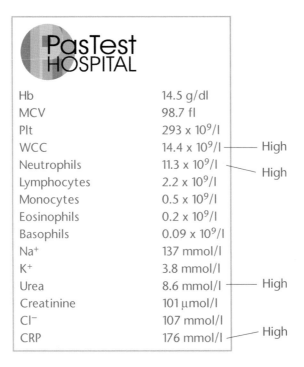

PasTest
HOSPITAL

Hb	14.5 g/dl
MCV	98.7 fl
Plt	293 x 10⁹/l
WCC	14.4 x 10⁹/l ——— High
Neutrophils	11.3 x 10⁹/l ～ High
Lymphocytes	2.2 x 10⁹/l
Monocytes	0.5 x 10⁹/l
Eosinophils	0.2 x 10⁹/l
Basophils	0.09 x 10⁹/l
Na⁺	137 mmol/l
K⁺	3.8 mmol/l
Urea	8.6 mmol/l ——— High
Creatinine	101 μmol/l
Cl⁻	107 mmol/l
CRP	176 mmol/l ——— High

1. From the initial investigations one should have identified the following:

- There is a raised WCC (predominantly comprising neutrophils), along with a raised CRP. The possibility of infection should be entertained.

- In addition, you will note a mildly raised urea, reflective of a mild degree of dehydration.

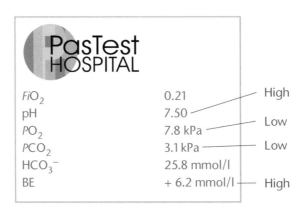

PasTest
HOSPITAL

FiO_2	0.21	High
pH	7.50	
PO_2	7.8 kPa	Low
PCO_2	3.1 kPa	Low
HCO_3^-	25.8 mmol/l	
BE	+ 6.2 mmol/l	High

2. The ABG features two findings:

- A low PaO_2. The patient is hypoxic. He has type 1 respiratory failure.

- A low $PaCO_2$. The patient is short of breath and hyperventilating, causing a low CO_2. This has led to a respiratory alkalosis.

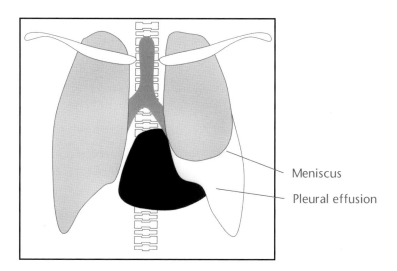

Meniscus

Pleural effusion

3. The chest X-ray indicates the likely cause for the findings so far.

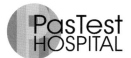

Radiology report

This is a PA chest X-ray of Captain John Boeing taken on 19 December 2005. He is a 54-year-old man. The technical quality of the film is ideal. The most striking finding is an area of radio-opacity on the left side of the chest from the lower zone extending to the mid-zone. The left hemi-diaphragm silhouette and the left costophrenic angle are not seen. A meniscus is noted at the lateral chest wall. No other pathology is noted on the film. These findings are in keeping with a moderate left-sided pleural effusion.

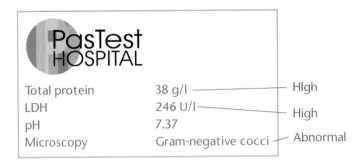

4. From the pleural fluid analysis one can see:

- This is an exudate with an elevated total protein and LDH level.

- Micro-organisms were identified in the form of Gram-negative cocci.

5. Putting all this information together and correlating it with the patient's clinical features, the likely cause for this pleural effusion is an underlying pneumonia. This is termed a parapneumonic pleural effusion.

The patient goes on to develop diarrhoea. The most likely cause is simple diarrhoea secondary to the commencement of antibiotics. However, one must be suspicious of *Clostridium difficile* as a causative organism for the diarrhoea, particularly since this patient has received a cephalosporin antibiotic.

The stool sample indicates the presence of *C. difficile* toxin. Ideally the causative antibiotic should be stopped and a suitable alternative used instead. Oral metronidazole should also be commenced to treat the *C. difficile*.

CASE SUMMARY

Pneumonia
Exudate pleural effusion (parapneumonic)
Type 1 respiratory failure with hyperventilation
Clostridium difficile infection (secondary to antibiotic treatment)

Case 111

DATA COVERED IN THIS CLINICAL CASE SCENARIO

- Biochemistry: U&E
- Endocrine: thyroid function tests
- Endocrine: short Synacthen® test
- Biochemistry: urinary electrolytes and osmolality

A 62-year-old male patient with inoperable lung cancer is admitted on the general medical take-in with acute confusion. Physical examination is unremarkable. Routine blood tests are sent, and the following results are obtained.

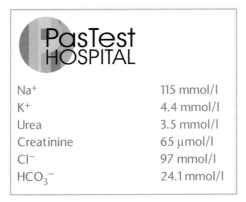

PasTest HOSPITAL	
Na⁺	115 mmol/l
K⁺	4.4 mmol/l
Urea	3.5 mmol/l
Creatinine	65 μmol/l
Cl⁻	97 mmol/l
HCO₃⁻	24.1 mmol/l

1. His weight is 61 kg. Estimate his glomerular filtration rate.

On the basis of these tests, a host of other investigations are organised. The results of these are shown below.

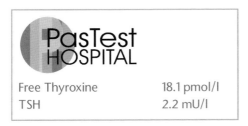

PasTest HOSPITAL	
Free Thyroxine	18.1 pmol/l
TSH	2.2 mU/l

2. What is his thyroid status?

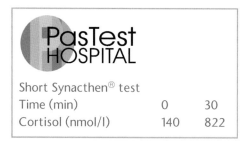

Short Synacthen® test

Time (min)	0	30
Cortisol (nmol/l)	140	822

3. **Interpret this test result.**

4. **His blood glucose is 4.6 mmol/l. Calculate his plasma osmolality.**

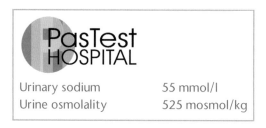

Urinary sodium	55 mmol/l
Urine osmolality	525 mosmol/kg

5. **What is the overall diagnosis?**

Answer 111

1. From the information given, the eGFR could be calculated (see page x for details). Alternatively, the following formula could be used to give an approximation of the GFR:

$$\text{Creatinine clearance} = \frac{(140 - 62) \times 61}{72 \times 65 \div 88.4} = 89.87 \text{ ml/min}$$

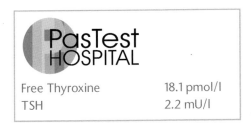

PasTest HOSPITAL	
Free Thyroxine	18.1 pmol/l
TSH	2.2 mU/l

2. His thyroid status is normal.

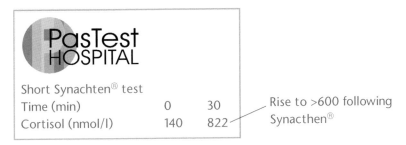

PasTest HOSPITAL

Short Synachten® test			
Time (min)	0	30	Rise to >600 following
Cortisol (nmol/l)	140	822	Synacthen®

3. This is a normal short Synacthen® test indicating normal adrenal gland function.

4. Plasma osmolality is calculated as:

Plasma osmolality = 2 x (115 + 4.4) + 3.5 + 4.6 = 246.9 mosmol/kg.

5. This patient fits the diagnostic criteria for SIADH, which is most likely secondary to his lung cancer, most commonly with the small cell subtype. His confusion is probably due to hyponatraemia.

CASE SUMMARY

Hyponatraemia
SIADH

Case 112

DATA COVERED IN THIS CLINICAL CASE SCENARIO

- Biochemistry: sweat analysis
- Genetics: mutation analysis
- Miscellaneous: PABA test
- Haematology: D-dimer
- Microbiology: sputum culture
- Miscellaneous: audiogram

A 28-year-old patient is admitted to hospital on account of weight loss. She has an inherited condition. Browsing through old medical notes, the admitting doctor noted the following results.

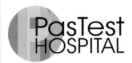

PasTest
HOSPITAL

Sweat analysis
112 mg sweat collected
Cl⁻   67 mmol/l
Na⁺   101 mmol/l
Genetics laboratory
ΔF508 mutation on long arm of chromosome 7

1. **What genetic condition does this patient have, and what is the inheritance pattern?**

The medical team are concerned about pancreatic exocrine insufficiency and organise a PABA test. The following result is returned.

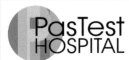

PasTest
HOSPITAL

PABA test
45% of oral PABA dose excreted in the urine

2. **Does the patient have pancreatic exocrine insufficiency?**

During the course of her inpatient stay, the patient develops a cough with a degree of haemoptysis. The SHO is concerned about the possibility of a pulmonary embolism, and requests the following test urgently.

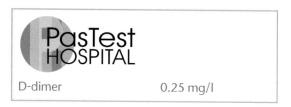

PasTest HOSPITAL	
D-dimer	0.25 mg/l

3. How does the D-dimer result help in managing the patient?

The patient then becomes pyrexic, and clinical signs suggest pneumonia. The medical team commence co-amoxiclav. Sputum is sent for culture. Two days later the following result is obtained.

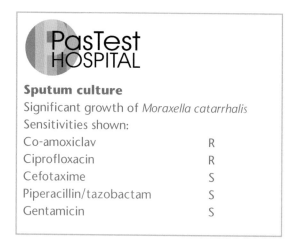

PasTest HOSPITAL

Sputum culture
Significant growth of *Moraxella catarrhalis*
Sensitivities shown:

Co-amoxiclav	R
Ciprofloxacin	R
Cefotaxime	S
Piperacillin/tazobactam	S
Gentamicin	S

On the basis of these sensitivities, and a worsening clinical state, the patient's antibiotics are changed to gentamicin.

A short time later the patient complains of hearing loss. The following audiogram is obtained.

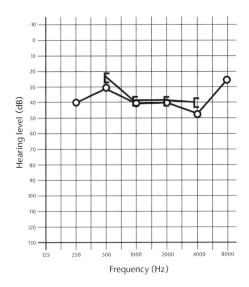

4. **What type of hearing loss has she developed, and how would you explain it?**

Answer 112

1. This patient has cystic fibrosis, which is inherited in an autosomal recessive manner.

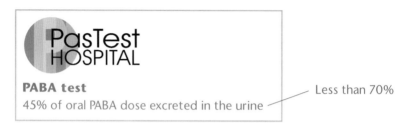

PABA test

45% of oral PABA dose excreted in the urine ⟶ Less than 70%

2. Yes. Pancreatic insufficiency is common in cystic fibrosis. More than 70% of the oral PABA should normally be excreted in the urine.

3. The D-dimer is normal. This indicates a very low probability of a thrombo-embolic event such as a pulmonary embolism. Other causes of haemoptysis should be sought. In very rare situations, the D-dimer can be normal in the presence of thrombosis, so clinical judgement is always essential when interpreting this result.

4. The audiogram shows sensorineural deafness. This is a rare but characteristic side-effect of aminoglycoside antimicrobials such as gentamicin.

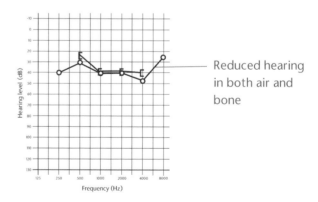

Reduced hearing in both air and bone

CASE SUMMARY

Cystic fibrosis
Pancreatic exocrine insufficiency
Pneumonia
Gentamicin-induced hearing loss

Case 113

DATA COVERED IN THIS CLINICAL CASE SCENARIO

- Haematology: full blood picture
- Haematology: haematinics
- Haematology: blood film
- Miscellaneous: CLO test
- Pathology: biopsy result

A 72-year-old man presents with increasing epigastric discomfort. He has been troubled with heartburn for several years. He admits to drinking 'more than he should'. The admitting doctor noted pallor, and requested the following.

PasTest
HOSPITAL

Hb	7.7 g/dl
MCV	69.5 fl
Plt	$512 \times 10^9/l$
WCC	$8.7 \times 10^9/l$
Serum iron	5 µmol/l
Ferritin	9 µg/l
TIBC	95 µmol/l
Vitamin B_{12}	265 ng/l
Folate	12.3 µg/l

1. How would you interpret these results?

A blood film is examined. The following report is obtained.

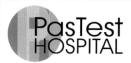

PasTest
HOSPITAL

Hypochromic, microcytic cells
Poikilocytosis and anisochromia
Occasional pencil cells seen

2. Is this result in keeping with your answer to question one?

He proceeds to have an oesophago-gastro-duodenoscopy (OGD). Two
abnormalities are noted. First, he is noted to have an abnormal appearance of
the lower oesophagus. Second, gastritis is observed. A biopsy is taken from the
lower oesophagus and the stomach. A CLO test is performed. You note the
following after 24 h.

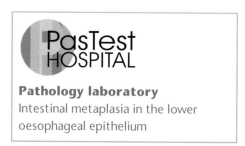

Pink circle

3. What treatment should be commenced on the basis of this CLO result?

One week later, the following result is phoned through from the pathology
laboratory:

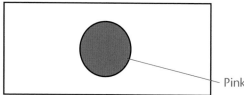

PasTest
HOSPITAL

Pathology laboratory
Intestinal metaplasia in the lower
oesophageal epithelium

4. What is the condition affecting the oesophagus?

CASES

Answer 113

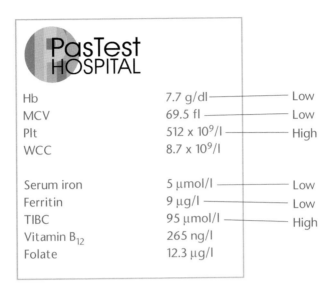

PasTest HOSPITAL

Hb	7.7 g/dl	Low
MCV	69.5 fl	Low
Plt	512 x 10⁹/l	High
WCC	8.7 x 10⁹/l	
Serum iron	5 μmol/l	Low
Ferritin	9 μg/l	Low
TIBC	95 μmol/l	High
Vitamin B₁₂	265 ng/l	
Folate	12.3 μg/l	

1. This patient has a microcytic anaemia. The mild thrombocytosis may be due to active bleeding. The haematinics show iron deficiency.

2. Yes. The abnormal blood cells described can all be found with iron deficiency.

3. The result is CLO positive, indicating gastric infection with *Helicobacter pylori*. The patient should be commenced on a course of antibiotics with a proton pump inhibitor, in an attempt to eradicate the infection.

4. The patient has Barrett's oesophagus, and will require surveillance OGDs for monitoring the disease.

CASE SUMMARY

Iron deficiency anaemia
Helicobacter pylori-positive gastritis
Barrett's oesophagus

Case 114

An 85-year-old male smoker is admitted complaining of abdominal discomfort. No abnormalities are detected on clinical examination, but some routine blood tests are requested. Your colleague is concerned about the following test result, and asks for your help.

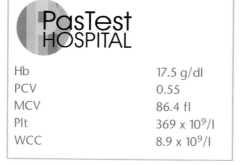

PasTest
HOSPITAL

Hb	17.5 g/dl
PCV	0.55
MCV	86.4 fl
Plt	369 x 10^9/l
WCC	8.9 x 10^9/l

1. What is this abnormality called, and how would you proceed?

The result is repeated and confirmed. He proceeds to have an estimation of red cell mass.

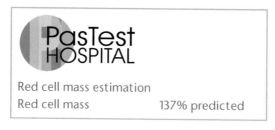

PasTest
HOSPITAL

Red cell mass estimation
Red cell mass   137% predicted

2. What does this result indicate?

On the basis of this result, arterial blood gas analysis was performed when the patient was breathing room air.

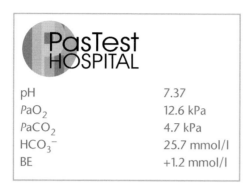

pH	7.37
PaO_2	12.6 kPa
$PaCO_2$	4.7 kPa
HCO_3^-	25.7 mmol/l
BE	+1.2 mmol/l

3. How would you interpret the blood gas?

An ultrasound scan of the abdomen revealed a mass in keeping with a renal cell carcinoma.

The patient proceeded to surgery, and underwent a nephrectomy. He spent 2 days in the intensive care unit after the operation, but returned to the ward on day 3 after the operation. His urine output deteriorated on day 4, and a urine specimen was sent for analysis.

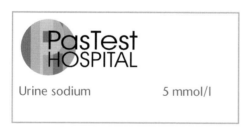

Urine sodium	5 mmol/l

4. What does this result tell you about the cause of the oliguria, and how would you treat the patient?

The patient's urine output recovers. Several days later he complains of a burning pain on passing urine, and of having to run to the toilet more often than normal. The following result is obtained on urinalysis.

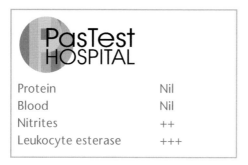

PasTest
HOSPITAL

Protein	Nil
Blood	Nil
Nitrites	++
Leukocyte esterase	+++

5. How would you interpret the urinalysis, and what further urine test would you request?

Answer 114

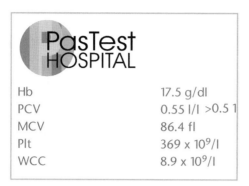

PasTest HOSPITAL	
Hb	17.5 g/dl
PCV	0.55 l/l >0.5 1
MCV	86.4 fl
Plt	369 x 10⁹/l
WCC	8.9 x 10⁹/l

1. The PCV is elevated, indicating polycythaemia. A measurement of the red cell mass is required to distinguish true polycythaemia from apparent polycythaemia.

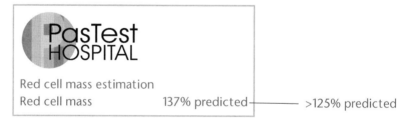

PasTest HOSPITAL

Red cell mass estimation
Red cell mass   137% predicted ———— >125% predicted

2. The red cell mass result indicates true polycythaemia, and a cause should be sought.

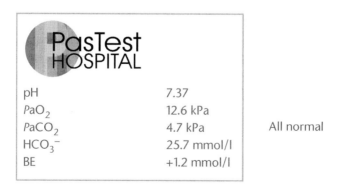

PasTest HOSPITAL		
pH	7.37	
PaO_2	12.6 kPa	
$PaCO_2$	4.7 kPa	All normal
HCO_3^-	25.7 mmol/l	
BE	+1.2 mmol/l	

3. The arterial blood gas analysis is entirely normal.

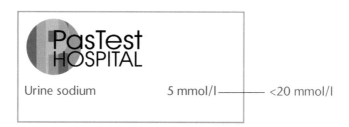

4. The urinary sodium concentration is low, suggesting that the oliguria is due to pre-renal causes, ie hypovolaemia. The patient requires intra-venous fluid resuscitation.

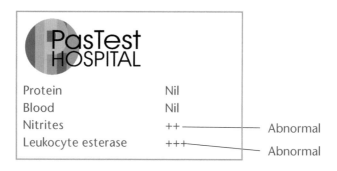

5. The urine contains nitrites and leukocyte esterase. In keeping with the clinical history, these changes are most commonly caused by a urinary tract infection. The most useful next investigation would be a urine culture.

CASE SUMMARY

Renal cell carcinoma
Postoperative pre-renal uraemia
Urinary tract infection

INDEX

Page numbers in **bold** refer to the clinical cases.